Younger People with Dementia

of related interest

Hearing the Voice of Older People with Dementia
Opportunities and Obstacles
Malcolm Goldsmith
ISBN 1 85302 406 6

Working with Carers
Christine Heron
ISBN 1 85302 562 3

Quality of Life
Philip Seed and Greg Lloyd
ISBN 1 85302 413 9

Caring for People in the Community
The New Welfare
Edited by Michael Titterton
ISBN 1 85302 112 1

Staff Supervision in a Turbulent Environment
Managing Process and Task in Front-line Services
Lynette Hughes and Paul Pengelly
ISBN 1 85302 327 2

Younger People with Dementia

Planning, Practice and Development

Edited by Sylvia Cox and John Keady

Foreword by Mary Marshall

Jessica Kingsley Publishers
London and Philadelphia

Acknowledgement is made to Robyn Yale for permission to reprint from *Developing Support Groups for Individuals with Early-Stage Alzheimer's Disearse: Planning, Implementation and Evaluation,* published by Health Professions Press (Baltimore, MD, USA). Copyright © 1995 by Robyn Yale. All rights reserved.

First published in the United Kingdom in 1999 by
Jessica Kingsley Publishers Ltd
116 Pentonville Road,
London N1 9JB,
England
and
325 Chestnut Street,
Philadelphia, PA 19106,
USA.

www.jkp.com

Second impression 1999

Copyright © 1999 Jessica Kingsley Publishers

Library of Congress Cataloging in Publication Data
A CIP catalog record for this book is available from the Library of Congress

British Library Cataloguing in Publication Data
Younger people with dementia: planning, practice and development
1.Dementia 2.Young adults - Mental health
I.Cox, Sylvia, 1948– II.Keady, John, 1961–
362.1'9683

ISBN 1 85302 588 7

Printed and Bound in Great Britain by
Athenaeum Press, Gateshead, Tyne and Wear

Contents

Acknowledgements

Many people have provided advice and support at various stages. In particular we would like to thank Professor Mary Marshall for encouragement to pursue the idea of the book; Ruhi Behi, Director of Post Registration Studies, School of Nursing and Midwifery Studies, University of Wales, Bangor for time in allowing John Keady to work on the book and to travel to Glasgow; Emeritus Professor Bill MacLennan for his valuable comments and advice, particularly on medical aspects; Irene Anderson for her objective comments; and Margaret Hope for her selfless dedication to duty in preparing and coordinating the manuscripts for this book.

This book is dedicated to Terry, Sara and Jennifer Cox and to Claire, Jessica and Christopher Keady.

Foreword

The authors kindly acknowledge my help in encouraging them to pursue the idea. All I did was share my view that this was a neglected field which needed an authoritative book. I was, of course, confident that the two authors were uniquely well placed to edit such a book. Whilst still employed by Strathclyde Regional Council, Sylvia Cox wrote the Dementia Services Development Centre a think piece on the policy and practice issues around services for younger people with dementia (Cox 1991). She was at the time responsible for planning services for people with dementia and was concerned that younger people and their families were falling through the net. With characteristic vigour she set about learning about the difficulties they face. When she came to work for the Dementia Services Development Centre it seemed sensible that she should build on this expertise. At the same time John Keady was undertaking research in North Wales in which he talked to younger people and their relatives. He too was reading widely and learning from a range of experts. Both are frantically busy people and, with this book, prove the axiom that if you want something done, you ask a busy person.

This is a neglected issue for several reasons. The numbers are not great, especially when compared with the huge numbers of older people with dementia. They are also people with complex and very different kinds of dementia, as this book demonstrates. Only a minority have Alzheimer's disease alone; much larger numbers have Alzheimer's disease related to learning disability or alcohol abuse, for example. We have, however, little idea of the actual numbers, since for many people dementia is a consequence of another disability or illness but not an inevitable consequence.

The causes are complex and so is the impact on their lives. This book provides very helpful insights into the repercussions of the diseases through every aspect of the lives of younger people with dementia and their families.

Less palatable reasons perhaps for the neglect of the issue are that some of the younger people with these diseases can be seen to have inflicted it on themselves through unsafe sex or alcohol abuse, and that for a whole set of reasons these are people who do not have much political or media clout. In part, because of their diversity and the small numbers, they are not organised into vocal organisations through which they speak or which speak on their behalf.

The fact that dementia is often a consequence of a range of diseases and disabilities presents considerable problems in the sense that there has been little cross-flow of expertise to and from the world of dementia care. Staff, for example, from the field of learning difficulties rarely meet staff from psychogeriatric specialisms. The way to deal with this is, of course, to be person-centred rather than preoccupied with diagnosis, but this is not easy. This book makes the case for a more person-centred style of care, and acknowledges that it is a real challenge when expertise and resources are in such short supply.

The book is an early step in collecting and making available knowledge and expertise in this field – a second, third and further steps are urgently required. It should raise expectations of what can be done and what needs to be done. Expertise and good practice are too patchy, but developing fast. The task is to continue the good work of the editors and chapter authors in order to try to minimise the anguish of individuals and families living with these conditions.

Professor Mary Marshall
Director, Dementia Services Development Centre

Introduction

Sylvia Cox and John Keady

This book is about dementia in younger people, which we define as being anyone under the age of 65 years, and those particularly in their 3rd, 4th, 5th, or 6th decade of life. Whilst recognising that in itself this is an arbitrary dividing line, and perpetuates ageist assumptions, we believe that this statement is necessary in order to redress the present inequitable balance in service provision and funding.

The seeds for this edited volume were sown in early 1994 when the authors met for the first time at the tenth Alzheimer's Disease International (ADI) conference in autumn 1994. That year the ADI conference was held in the tranquil and inspiring surroundings of the University of Edinburgh. Perhaps seduced by the academic surroundings, and flushed with the success of recent publications on the area of 'younger onset dementia' – some of which are cited in this volume – we mulled over thoughts of 'doing something together' on the subject. One of our thoughts was to try and publish an edited volume dedicated solely to the subject of younger people with dementia. Nothing concrete happened for a couple of years until April 1996, when Sylvia and the Dementia Services Development Centre hosted a one-day conference on 'Younger People with Dementia'. The conference set an interesting programme and took a multidisciplinary approach which drew contributors from across the United Kingdom. The afternoon workshops at the conference were one of the successes and covered the following topics:

- Commissioning and purchasing a comprehensive service.
- Person-centred planning for younger people with dementia.
- A balance of care for younger people with dementia.
- Setting quality standards.
- The pros and cons of specialist and integrated services.

Participation in the dissemination and analysis of the workshops rekindled our energy and this book is a consequence of that commitment. Indeed, the format of the workshops bear more than a passing resemblance to the structure of this book.

On the whole, services for younger people with dementia, save for some notable exceptions, are rare and those that do exist have been built up from the enthusiasm and dedication of staff and carers who have ploughed a furrow through the intricacies of health and social care funding. Younger people with dementia and their carers demand a more focused and coordinated agenda, which builds upon the framework set out in the Health Advisory Services (HAS) report *Mental Health Services: Heading for Better Care* (Health Advisory Service 1996). To make a reality out of this report title requires considerable attention and debate. Whilst we do not pretend that this book is an end in itself, it does, perhaps, represent a small step towards this ideal.

About the book

The book embraces medical, sociological and psychological approaches to the understanding of younger onset dementia, as well as including more subjective encounters with carers and younger people with dementia themselves. The book has been divided into four sections which encompass a range of academic, planning and practice perspectives and we will now briefly rehearse the contents of each section.

Part One has been named 'Setting the Scene' and includes four separate but interrelated chapters. The first is by Jane McLennan who introduces a medical practitioner's approach to assessment and service response issues whilst reviewing some of the investigations undertaken to establish a diagnostic understanding. Kirstie Woodburn then explores the epidemiological aspects of younger onset dementia which is based on her own studies in the Lothian area of Scotland. The next chapter by Gregor McWalter and James Chalmers provides an overview of the intricacies of needs assessment and its implication for younger people with dementia and their carers. Finally, in this section, Sylvia Cox explores the wider policy and planning perspectives and the need for an inclusive approach based on person-centred values.

In Part Two, 'Specific Considerations' appertaining to younger people with dementia are covered and four separate conditions are discussed. First, Steve Jamieson sets out the implications of HIV-related brain impairment. Second, Roseanne Cetnarskyj and Mary Porteous describe the particular issues relating to Huntington's disease and the practical implications for staff. Third, Sally-Ann Cooper sets out the clinical picture for people with learning disabilities and dementia and some of the service implications. Fourth, Simon Crowe provides an overview of alcohol-related dementia based on his research and practical involvement in service development in Victoria, Australia.

Part Three draws together a number of strands which embrace the area of 'Developing an Individual Understanding'; this is presented from both a personal, subjective viewpoint and within a family care context. The first chapter in this section is written by John Killick and presents his experiences of talking with younger people and their relatives in a variety of settings. Diane Seddon then goes on to explore the employment issues for caregivers and also presents a range of transitional coping strategies which have implications for both employers and professionals. Jane Gilliard tackles the emotive subject of young people in their teenage years who are involved in a caring experience. John Keady and Mike Nolan provide an overview of the care giving experience and the service implications this entails. Gretta Peachment closes the section with a discussion of environmental and design issues for younger people in continuing care, an area which has received little attention.

Part Four addresses 'Practice Developments' and opens with a review of interventions available for younger people and their carers by Bob Woods. Robyn Yale then builds upon this contribution by specifying a model of group work with younger people in the early stages of dementia. Next, Alan Chapman highlights the importance of education and training for practitioners involved in all aspects of dementia care. The book ends with Sylvia Cox and John Keady setting out some of the challenges that lie ahead.

Terminology used in the book

The language used to refer to younger people with dementia will vary during this book. We have attempted to promote the term 'younger people', although the traditional medical definition for describing dementia acquired by people aged 65 and under is 'presenile' and/or 'early onset dementia', the latter being stated in both the ICD-10 (World Health Organization 1993) and the DSM-IV (American Psychiatric Association 1994) classification. Whilst our personal preference is to use the descriptive terms 'younger onset' and 'younger people with dementia', chapter authors may, from time to time, revert to using terminology such as 'early onset dementia'. Where this is retained in the text, the terminology is set within the author's preference, professional approach or research context, or in citation from secondary literature sources. However, whatever language is used, the principle aims of this book remain the same:

1. To inform readers about the extent and nature of dementia in younger people in a way that is accessible to a wide range of policy makers, planners and practitioners in relevant fields.

2. To explore and promote policy and practice perspectives from the point of view of users and carers.

3. To explore the meaning of needs assessment from the individual and planning perspectives.

4. To present a range of policy planning and practice approaches which emphasise multidisciplinary working.

References

Astute readers will notice that certain references are repeated during the text. We would like to think that this is not a shortcoming of the editors, but presents the reality of too few studies in this field. Hopefully, this position will be rectified as the years ahead unfold.

Case studies

Case studies are provided in many of the chapters. Their use is not only to illustrate key points but also to use real-life situations as a learning and training resource. Where case studies are provided, care has been taken to preserve the anonymity of the person(s) involved by changing names, places and other identifying information.

Exclusions from the book

Whilst we thought it important to highlight the range of conditions which might involve younger people with dementia, we have consciously chosen to exclude those such as acquired brain injury, secondary dementias such as Parkinson's disease, and the rarer forms of dementia. This is not to imply that we are unsympathetic to people with these conditions, rather it reflects the complexities of the situation, especially on the boundaries of progressive/nonprogressive cognitive impairment and physical disability.

Sylvia Cox and John Keady
January 1998

PART ONE

Setting the Scene

CHAPTER I

Assessment and Service Responses for Younger People with Dementia
A Medical Overview

Jane McLennan

Preface

As a psychiatrist working for the last eight years in a range of hospital/clinic settings, including a memory clinic, I have tried to give an account of the complexities of assessment and service issues involved without totally overwhelming the lay reader with technicalities and jargon. This is a difficult balance and medical colleagues will appreciate the limitations such simplification entails.

The case studies, appropriately anonymised, are drawn from my clinical work in multidisciplinary assessment and in extensive experience of sharing the diagnosis. My knowledge and understanding of younger onset dementia has been enhanced by learning from colleagues in a range of other professions and not least from the patients and families I have known over the years.

My association with both the Dementia Services Development Centre and Alzheimer Scotland – Action on Dementia has widened my understanding of the broader dementia issues, particularly in relation to the need for collaborative working and joint commissioning between health, social work and the voluntary sector and the importance of involving those who use services and those who care for them.

Introduction

Dementia is a syndrome describing a characteristic pattern of symptoms and signs caused by a number of different disease processes. They are usually caused by the death of cells in critical areas of the brain which cause impairment in memory, reduced ability to learn new material and deficiency in judgement, language and abstract thinking. There may also be signs of mood disturbance, personality change and disordered behaviour. Such abnormalities affect and often disrupt everyday living, work and the social life of relatives. Dementia has been defined as:

> A syndrome due to disease of the brain, usually of a chronic or progressive nature in which there is an impairment of multiple higher cortical functions, including memory, thinking, orientation, comprehension, calculation, learning capacity, language and judgement. Consciousness is not clouded. The cognitive impairments are commonly accompanied and occasionally preceded by deterioration in emotional control, social behaviour or motivation. (World Health Organization 1993)

It should be emphasised that if a disease causes dementia early in life it affects clinical progression of the illness. This combines with family dynamics and personality to create unique experiences and issues for people with younger onset dementia, their carers and families. In particular, younger people with dementia are observed as experiencing:

- decline in short-term memory
- symptoms of anxiety and/or depression
- personality change with blunting of emotional perception and responsiveness
- lack of interest in and withdrawal from normal activities including family relationships
- forgetting appointments
- inability to perform routine tasks to the same standard as previously
- poor concentration
- word-finding difficulties
- repetitive conversation
- the development, at times, of paranoid ideas.

Usually it is the person closest who notices these changes first, but in the very early stages the person with dementia may also feel that 'something is wrong'. It is often a very bewildering and frightening experience. People with subtle, early changes of dementia, are often aware of these experiences but are unable to understand what they are. Complaints of physical illness can be quite common at this time together with headaches, feelings of 'not being quite right' and excessive concern for other aspects of physical health (see also Keady 1997).

Progressive or treatable forms of dementia

Alzheimer's disease is the most common cause of dementia, followed by Lewy Body disease, mixed vascular dementia/Alzheimer's disease and the vascular dementias. These three types of dementia are thought to make up approximately 90 per cent of all causes in the developed world. With current modes of therapy, all are irreversible.

Treatable conditions include vitamin B12 deficiency and normal pressure hydrocephalus. One of the key tasks of health care services is to distinguish progressive from treatable dementia. An overview of both these conditions will now follow.

Irreversible causes of dementia

DEGENERATIVE DEMENTIAS

Alzheimer's disease

This is probably the commonest cause (50%) of all dementias. It has a gradual and insidious onset, which may be mistaken for depression, anxiety, or normal ageing. It has a relentlessly progressive course. Memory, daily living skills and comprehension normally decline globally, and it is more common in women.

Lewy Body disease

This was first described some decades ago, and has been the subject of intense research over the past few years (McKeith *et al.* 1994). Hallucinations, delusions, mood disturbance and fluctuation in the level of awareness are common features. Excessive sensitivity to neuroleptic drugs (i.e. drugs commonly used to treat major mental illness and behavioural disturbances in dementia such as chlorpromazine, haloperidol, thioridazine) is another characteristic feature. The disease normally has a much more rapid progression, and death frequently follows within one to two years after diagnosis. It is said to account for up to 20 per cent of dementia cases (Perry *et al.*1990).

Pick's disease

This is a rare condition which affects the frontal and temporal lobes in the brain (Alzheimer's disease characteristically affects the parietal and temporal lobes). It usually has a gradual onset, with deterioration in personality and behaviour more prominent than poor memory for recent events. Selective problems involving disinhibition and speech disturbances are prominent. There are also marked mood changes which include shallowness, lack of concern and emotional lability. The age of onset is usually before 60 years.

Frontal dementias

Clinically often indistinguishable from Pick's disease, the presentation is one of marked personality change, social disinhibition, incongruity of mood, and impairment of speech. Short-term memory and visuospatial orientation are relatively preserved. There is often a family history of a similar dementia (50% of those affected have a parent with dementia, Gustafson 1987). An accurate diagnosis is usually only made at post mortem.

Huntington's disease

Dementia is usually a late manifestation of Huntington's disease, but people with the disease commonly develop dementia-type symptoms before the age of 65 years. Disorders of movement, paranoid ideas (concerns that others are against one, or a belief that important events are connected to one), depression, and non-memory signs of dementia are usually particularly prominent in this condition (see also Chapter 6).

Parkinson's disease

Twenty to thirty per cent of people with Parkinson's disease develop dementia, usually late in the disease (Marder *et al.* 1995) with clinical features of subcortical damage. This includes poor concentration, inability to plan actions and thoughts, slowness of thinking, indecisiveness, and apathy. These are more prominent than short-term memory loss in the early stages.

VASCULAR DEMENTIA

Vascular dementia (i.e. dementia caused by strokes) is more common in men, mainly due to the higher risk factors for cardiovascular disease in men rather than women. It is characterised by a sudden onset with stepwise deterioration, relating to episodes of further strokes. There is often a past history of hypertension, ischaemic heart disease or peripheral vascular disease. People with this type of dementia normally have a patchy loss of ability and cognitive functioning, they often have relative preservation of their personality, but a prominent loss of short-term memory. There are many subtypes of vascular dementia, well described in a review by Amar and Wilcock (1996).

INFECTIOUS DEMENTIAS

Syphilis

Dementia is a late feature of syphilis, emerging decades after the initial infection. The disease process affects the frontal lobes particularly, leading to marked personality change and disinhibition. Antibiotic treatment can stop deterioration, but not reverse it. It is much less common in Western Europe and North America than it was 50 or more years ago.

Prion dementia

These are a group of diseases causing 'spongiform encephalopathy' a condition in which the brain has a sponge-like appearance at post mortem. These diseases were previously called slow virus diseases, but it is now clear that the transmissible agent is a subviral protein particle called a 'prion'. It can be acquired by the transfer of infected material between humans (e.g. organ transplants and human growth hormone treatment), or very rarely may be inherited in some families (15% of Creutzfeldt-Jakob disease (CJD) cases are familial: see Collinge et al. 1990). CJD and Gerstmann-Straussler syndrome are examples of this group of dementias. There is no hard evidence that animals infected with bovine spongiform encephalopathy can transmit these diseases to humans, although further research still needs to be conducted in this area (Rossor 1996; Will et al. 1996).

MECHANICAL DEMENTIAS

This group consists of:

- subdural haematoma
- normal pressure hydrocephalus
- tumour.

All of the above will be briefly outlined (see below) and if not detected sufficiently early and treated, often lead on to dementia.

METABOLIC AND ENDOCRINE DEMENTIAS

Thyroid disease

Chronic hypothyroidism may produce a dementia associated with features of depression and slowness. An underactive thyroid is relatively common in older people and hypothyroidism may occur alongside a dementia. Hypothyroidism is often misdiagnosed as a feature of old age or depression. It is vitally important, therefore, that biochemical tests for hypothyroidism are organised in such cases. Treatment with replacement therapy corrects thyroxin deficiency, but has no effect on the coincidental dementia unless this is the primary cause.

Vitamin deficiency

The most common vitamin deficiency to be associated with mental impairment in this country is a lack of the vitamin thiamine associated with chronic alcoholism. In addition to dementia there is weakness of the muscles involved in eye movements, an unsteadiness and muscle weakness, and loss of sensation in the limbs due to peripheral nerve damage. A similar picture was sometimes observed several decades ago in pregnant women with severe morning sickness (hyperemesis gravidarum). Deficiency of folic acid or vitamin B12 can cause dementia in old age, but is rarely a problem in younger individuals.

TOXIC DEMENTIAS

Chronic alcohol toxicity

The relationship between chronic alcohol dependence and the development of dementia is probably a much more complex one than simple vitamin deficiency. This is an area which requires further exploration. See Chapter 8 for more detailed information.

Liver and kidney disease

These are disorders of the body's ability to store certain elements, causing abnormal deposition of substances, for example Wilson's disease, where copper is abnormally deposited in the liver, brain and eyes.

Heavy metal poisoning

An example is lead, although this is now extremely rare.

Reversible or pseudo-dementias: differential diagnosis

These conditions, by definition, are disorders which may be mistaken for a dementing illness but are in fact reversible. Their recognition and treatment can lead to a return to normal cognitive functioning. Assessment can be problematic in patients from ethnic and cultural minorities and it is important that health care professionals take into account and respond to the needs of each individual and seek assistance if there are communication problems. The earlier a possible dementing illness is identified, the earlier an accurate diagnosis can be made. Treatment can slow, halt or reverse the progression of the disorder. Conditions in this category are as follows:

DEPRESSION

This is probably the commonest condition to be mistaken for an early dementing illness, particularly in those families in which another member has had dementia, and where suspicion of a diagnosis of dementia may be particularly high.

Common symptoms of depression include poor concentration, forgetfulness, paucity of thoughts, anxiety, flattening of emotions and lack of emotional responsiveness. Lack of motivation and narrowing of interests are common in both depression and early dementia. In families who have already experienced younger onset dementia, people with depression often mistake their symptoms as the onset of a dementing illness and can, as a consequence, delay seeking treatment. Depression is also a very common condition and can, with careful and appropriate treatment, be successfully treated, as illustrated in Case study 1.

Case study 1: Mrs P

Mrs P was a 40-year-old lady who was married with two young children. She approached her GP requesting referral for further investigation of her memory, as she was afraid that she was beginning to suffer from dementia. During the course of the interview, she revealed that her mother had developed Alzheimer's disease when Mrs P was aged nine. The diagnosis was made when Mrs P was in her late teens, and her mother died when Mrs P was in her 20s. During the period before diagnosis, Mrs P and her family had to cope with their mother's deteriorating memory, and her inability to care for the family in her normal manner. They experienced her changing personality and altered emotional responsiveness, and her inability to fulfil her role as a parent. It was in some ways an enormous relief to the family when Mrs P's mother was diagnosed as suffering from dementia, but by that time she was very unwell, and required institutional care for the last five years of her life.

Mrs P had lived with the fear that she would also develop Alzheimer's disease. Once her children were born, she was very afraid that she would not be able to care for them as she wanted to, and that they would go through the same traumas and profound losses that she had done. She was also very concerned for her husband, not wishing him to have to cope as 'a lone parent' and look after her.

Over the last three years Mrs P had been concerned that she was suffering from dementia, and had finally been persuaded by her husband

---

to see her GP. At interview, Mrs P gave a history of poor memory for recent events, forgetfulness, feeling tired all the time, lack of emotional responsiveness, irritability and finding it difficult to cope with her day-to-day activities. She felt that she was failing both as a wife and mother. Combined with this, she felt that her self-care and her care of her children, husband and home had also deteriorated. These symptoms had been present and had fluctuated to a greater or lesser degree since the birth of her first child seven years ago.

On investigation Mrs P was, in fact, suffering from a chronic post-natal depression which had had a relapsing and remitting course over the years and had been particularly bad for the past six months. She was very relieved to be diagnosed as suffering from depression rather than dementia, and it was explained to her that should her cognitive functioning not return to normal once her depression was treated, then her memory should be investigated further.

Mrs P made a full recovery some three months after beginning treatment and her fears regarding younger onset dementia have diminished considerably.

THYROID DISEASE

Chronic hypothyroidism may produce dementia-like features with depression and slowness, poor concentration and a poor recent memory. With treatment these symptoms usually disappear.

NORMAL PRESSURE HYDROCEPHALUS

People with this disorder present with a triad of characteristic symptoms, namely dementia, disturbance of walking and balance and urinary incontinence out of keeping with the degree of cognitive decline. This is caused by increased fluid in the brain leading to pressure effects. The symptoms are fully reversible if it is detected and treated early enough.

SUBDURAL HAEMATOMA

This is usually the result of a head injury, and most commonly occurs in older people and in individuals with chronic alcohol dependency. A small clot develops external to the lining of the brain and slowly enlarges. Symptoms may develop over a period of hours, days, weeks or months with headache, confusion and often fluctuating level of consciousness being characteristic.

Sometimes stroke-like symptoms can develop. If the cause is recognised early and the clot evacuated, full recovery can ensue.

TUMOUR

Tumours within the brain can cause a dementia-like syndrome by increasing pressure within the brain. If the tumour is recognised and is not malignant, treatment may promote full recovery.

Diagnostic investigations

Most studies of younger onset dementia have shown that it is very rare to find a treatable condition other than depression (Ames, Flicker and Helme 1992; Ferran *et al.* 1996). Despite this, elucidating the diagnosis is of great importance in addressing current problems, exploring the likely course of the disease, and in planning future treatment, care and support. Careful history taking and examination, preferably within a multidisciplinary team, are still the basis upon which an accurate clinical diagnosis is made (Ferran *et al.* 1996; Verhey *et al.* 1993).

The following investigations are often used to aid in the diagnosis, and in skilled hands can be extremely useful.

Blood tests

These include a full blood count and thyroid function tests for signs of thyroid underactivity, and anaemia with low serum B12 and folate levels. These are usually routine screening tests, and may be useful in determining the general health of the individual.

Brain scans

There are many techniques used to look at the structure and function of the brain, such as the following.

COMPUTED TOMOGRAPHY (CT)

This involves taking X-ray 'slices' through the brain to show its structure. The CT scan findings will vary depending upon the condition experienced, for instance:

- *Alzheimer's disease* reveals a differential loss of volume from the medial temporal lobes compared with total brain volume

- *vascular dementia* demonstrates a picture of patchy loss of brain matter as a result of stroke, or small white matter lesions
- *subdural haematomas* show up as space occupying lesions between the brain and the skull
- *Pick's disease* and other frontal dementias reveal a very significant loss of frontal lobe volume compared with the volume of the rest of the brain
- *Normal pressure hydrocephalus* would be demonstrated by enlarged ventricles and fluid filled spaces and the volume of brain matter would be reduced
- *Alcohol related dementia* does not produce a consistent picture on CT scanning.

MAGNETIC RESONANCE IMAGING (MRI)

This is a much more lengthy procedure, normally taking 20 to 40 minutes. The machine makes a lot of noise which can be worrying. The person has to stay completely still, as any movement ruins the scan. MRI shows the structure of the brain in very fine detail and can be particularly useful in multi-infarct dementia where a CT scan may not pick up small infarcts.

MAGNETIC RESONANCE SPECTROSCOPY (MRS)

MRS shows the biochemical processes in the brain but, as yet, has added little to our knowledge of dementia.

SINGLE PHOTON EMISSION COMPUTED TOMOGRAPHY (SPECT SCANNING)

In SPECT scanning radioactive dye is injected into the patient's forearm, it is taken up into the brain and held for a minimum of 24 hours. The purpose of the scan is to demonstrate the blood supply to the brain by producing a 'contour map':

- *Alzheimer's disease* is demonstrated by differential reduction in the blood supply to the temporal and parietal lobes, and often with a reduction of blood supply to the frontal lobes
- *frontal dementias* are demonstrated by marked reduction of blood supply to the frontal lobes
- *vascular dementias* are demonstrated by patchy loss of blood supply to different areas of the brain.

POSITRON EMISSION TOMOGRAPHY (PET SCAN)

This is a very detailed scan demonstrating biochemical processes within the living brain. It is currently a research tool and requires very expensive equipment. At present it is a slow procedure and has added little to our knowledge of dementia so far.

ELECTROENCEPHALOGRAPHY (EEG)

This examines electrical activity within the brain. The procedure normally takes a minimum of 40 minutes to carry out, and many patients are unable to relax or stay still for a long enough period. The EEG can provide very helpful information in supporting the diagnoses of Alzheimer's disease and Huntington's disease, vascular and frontal dementias and CJD, as well as excluding the presence of a tumour. To embellish these points a little:

- *Alzheimer's disease* is associated with characteristic gross slowing of electrical activity over the temporal and parietal areas
- *frontal dementias* are associated with similar slowing over the frontal lobes, with relatively normal activity elsewhere
- *vascular dementia* and tumour display patches of abnormal electrical activity surrounding the areas of infarct or abnormal growth
- *Huntington's disease* characteristically produces a flat pattern of electrical activity.

LUMBAR PUNCTURE

This is a procedure whereby a small sample of cerebrospinal fluid which surrounds the brain and spinal cord is removed from the spinal column. It is normally only used in the diagnosis of unusual dementias, or when an infective cause is suspected.

Is early onset different from late onset dementia?

Many of the differences are caused by the different diseases causing the syndrome. It is believed by some that people with younger onset dementia have a more rapid deterioration than those with late onset dementia. This is not a consistent finding in the literature (Christie and Wood 1988; Lucca *et al.* 1993). It would seem that the severity of the disease at the time of the first contact rather than age at first contact is the more accurate determinant of survival and rate of progression (Haupt, Kurz and Pollmann 1992; Newens *et al.* 1993; Treves *et al.* 1986).

The question of why the needs of those with younger onset dementia differ from those who develop the syndrome in later life also deserves consideration (Alzheimer's Disease Society 1992a; Cox and McLennan 1994). One factor is that the person may still be in employment, and often is the main wage earner in the household. There will probably be the presence of a younger partner and family, and there may still be school-age children (Aldridge and Becker 1993). The family may well still be in a state of growth and flux within its life cycle, and there may still be parenting roles to fulfil. There is likely to be a greater degree of social disruption, and more people are involved in the caring network.

Previous studies have demonstrated that people with younger onset dementia may have a particularly high incidence of depression, anxiety and challenging behaviour. In the Liverpool sample (Ferran *et al.* 1996), almost half had experienced depression and almost one-third had symptoms of challenging behaviour. The high levels of psychiatric morbidity in this group are reflected in their high use of community and institutional services compared with people with late onset dementia (Baldwin 1994; Ferran *et al.* 1996; Newens, Forster and Kay 1995).

Younger onset dementia appears when most people still expect to be leading a healthy, active, independent life. Onset at a more active stage of life can have the effect of making problem behaviour seem more extreme. Their physical strength is also often greater. The secondary consequences of symptoms in younger onset dementia are often related to the tasks which may still be undertaken at this stage in life. For example, failure to recognise difficulties in planning, organisation, problem solving and memory are very likely to result in frustration, tension and anxiety. Wrong decisions can also have major repercussions for those still involved in work and business.

What may be regarded as a clinically early stage is often, in functional terms, potentially severely disabling if not managed positively. Imagine the extreme problems we would face in our daily lives if we were unable to learn new information, retrieve recent information, or remember the names of a range of objects or work colleagues.

Treatment issues

Treatment of dementia has become a much more topical issue in the realms of purchasers of health care as the prospect of effective drug treatment for Alzheimer's disease and vascular dementia is becoming a reality. Of course, those involved in the field of dementia care are well aware that there are many non-drug treatments and strategies available for the management of different aspects of the dementia syndrome, though they cannot affect the core biological processes causing the disease process. Social stimulation, psychological strategies and a positive emotional environment all have a very positive impact on the quality of life of the person with dementia and their partner and family. They may slow the progression of the disease and may effect an improvement in behaviour and function for a time.

Tacrine was the first drug treatment for Alzheimer's disease to be licensed in most countries of the world, and there has now been considerable research and evaluation of this drug. Its efficiency is marginal and limited by its toxicity. It was never licensed in Britain. At the time of writing, Donepezil hydrochloride (Aricept) is the first anti-Alzheimer drug to be licensed in Britain (Rogers *et al.* 1998), though its availability is patchy due to many health boards and authorities refusing to fund its use. In common with Tacrine, it is only mildly effective, but has few side effects and is generally well tolerated. This issue is discussed further by Bob Woods in Chapter 14.

Multidisciplinary assessment

GPs deal so infrequently with younger onset dementia that they are not usually expert in carrying out the extensive investigations required to establish a diagnosis, particularly where the cause is uncommon. However, they need to have sufficient knowledge to include rarer causes in the differential diagnosis for a patient's symptoms. Referral of the person with their partner / close relative to either a psychiatrist, a neurologist, or, if available, a memory clinic or specialist centre is recommended. This may be done either directly or via the community mental health team.

A multidisciplinary assessment is preferable (Ferran *et al.* 1996; Verhey *et al.* 1993). Where a memory clinic exists, people may find that this is a more acceptable means of having their memory problems investigated than being referred to a psychiatrist or neurologist alone. The ideal is a memory clinic integrated within a specialist younger onset dementia service. Memory clinics vary in their procedures and, though they have been widely described in the literature (Wright and Lindesay 1995), there are few examples of evaluation, in particular in relation to patients and carers attending such services (Ames, Flicker and Helme 1992; Ferran *et al.* 1996; McMurdo *et al.* 1993). There are over 20 clinics in the UK which provide services to people with memory and cognitive problems (Health Advisory Service (HAS) 1996). They are often attached to university academic departments as they are a focus for research and provide standardised evaluation of mental and physical disability. More general clinics run by neurologists, old age psychiatrists and neuropsychiatrists also evaluate memory and cognitive problems.

It is important that memory clinics do not function simply as a 'labelling service'. They should do more for the person with dementia and the carer than give the diagnosis. Counselling and ongoing support or care is essential. In an ideal situation, the memory clinic would be integrated with assessment and care management within social services and the delivery of care by the national health service. Evaluation could be an integral part of the whole service for people with younger onset dementia.

The organisation of a memory clinic is broadly as below (modified to take account of the age group). The core staff comprise:

- psychiatrist with special interest in dementia/responsibility for early onset service
- neurologist (geriatrician in over-65 service)
- neuropsychologist
- occupational therapist
- community psychiatric nurse
- specialist social worker
- physiotherapist available for referrals.

An assessment is usually carried out by each discipline, including home assessment if possible. Specialist radiological investigations and neuropsychological assessments may be carried out to establish areas of poor functioning in the brain and their consequences. Part of the general assessment and investigation should also focus on areas of good functioning and remaining new learning ability with a view to building upon these to maximise independence, self-esteem and quality of life.

Common medical investigations include:

- full blood count – checking for anaemia, low serum vitamin B12 and folate levels, and evidence of excessive alcohol consumption
- routine blood biochemistry – looking for treatable physical disease
- thyroid function tests.

These, along with clinical assessment, should exclude most treatable causes of mental impairment such as thyroid disease, depression, vitamin deficiency and toxic causes of dementia.

More specialised investigations may then be performed, for instance:

- CT scan to look at the structure of the brain
- MRI scan to look at the fine structure of the brain (may rarely be carried out instead of a CT scan)
- SPECT scan, if available, to examine the pattern of blood supply to the brain
- EEG to look for abnormal electrical activity in the brain, either globally or focally
- lumbar puncture may very rarely be carried out, to search for an infective cause.

Once the results of the team assessments have been discussed, a reasonably firm diagnosis can be reached.

Sharing the diagnosis

Once the diagnosis is made, good practice would dictate that it is shared with the person with dementia and their partner and/or family. Sometimes people do not wish to know the label of their illness, and sometimes deny it when it is given. In these situations, it is accepted that someone has the right not to have the diagnosis forced upon them (Fearnley *et al.* 1997). It is important to explain the cause of memory impairment and other cognitive, emotional and personality changes which occur as a consequence of disease processes in the brain. Often the knowledge that repetitive questioning or conversation, emotional changes, lack of care and concern, loss of skills, poor personal hygiene and poor recent memory are due to a disease process, and not wilful awkwardness, is a relief. The changes likely to occur in the future and the effects these will have on the person with younger onset dementia and their family need to be addressed sensitively, however, as it may be too over-whelming to look too far into the future at this stage (McGowin 1993).

Taking a problem-oriented approach is very helpful, and is realistically reassuring. Helping the person with dementia and their carer or close rela-tives to break the illness down into problems which can have a solution, rather than a progressive, degenerative disease, is a much more positive and helpful approach. If started early enough in the illness, it can help signifi-cantly to relieve stress.

Dementia also affects the family with whom the person lives. Carers pro-vide valuable social support and care and may ameliorate some of the effects of the cognitive impairments and so reduce the level of disability experi-

Case study 2: Mr and Mrs R

Mr R's GP had recently attended a training session on 'diagnosis and assessment in dementia'. Mr R had been brought to the surgery by his wife and daughter, who were concerned about his recent memory and changes in his personality. He was forgetting dates and appointments, and becoming careless and unconcerned about financial matters. They also noticed that he was becoming socially withdrawn, which was in complete contrast to his previous personality. Other relevant points were that he was an insulin dependent diabetic, and was only 62. His GP could not detect any memory problems at interview, but felt further investigation was indicated and so referred him to the memory clinic.

At the memory clinic, both Mr and Mrs R were seen together, and the history and examination confirmed the suspicion that he had an early dementia, which was probably of the Alzheimer type. Other investigations had to be performed, such as brain scans and a neuropsychological assessment, to confirm the diagnosis.

At the first interview, Mr R was clearly unconcerned about his memory problems, but Mrs R was very worried and stressed. It seemed sensible to discuss the likely diagnoses, and their implications, even though this was a very early stage in the assessment. The couple were invited back, along with their daughter, to discuss the results of the investigations at which stage the diagnosis of probable Alzheimer's disease was confirmed. The disease was explained, and put into the context of a series of problems, most of which had a workable solution. The likely course of the disease was discussed, and issues surrounding future care needs and support were explored. Legal and financial implications were also discussed. In many ways this was a relief to Mrs R. Mr R was relatively unaffected by the diagnosis. This was a reflection of his general lack of concern, and evidence of frontal lobe involvement in the disease process.

The couple were also seen by the community psychiatric nurse (CPN) and social worker for further counselling and support, as well as ongoing education about the disease. A CPN or social worker linked to a community mental health team would provide the benefit of a range of other professional support along with access to community services and ongoing monitoring and review. The problems of Mr R's short-term memory were tackled in a step-by-step manner, with practical solutions sought as far as possible. The couple were encouraged to restart some of their previous social activities, to be as open as they felt comfortable with regarding Mr R's memory problems, and to enlist the help and support of their friends and family.

enced. However, caring has social and health costs with carers often showing physical and mental health symptoms (such as exhaustion, depression, anxiety). It is, therefore, extremely important that the health care needs of carers and families are monitored and addressed, whether or not the younger person with dementia is receiving specialist mental health care. These issues are exemplified in the following two case studies.

Key points

- Raising awareness of the GP that complaints of mild memory problems are a legitimate cause for concern and need prompt action, especially in younger people.

- The family noticed the problems first. Although they appeared rather insubstantial in medical terms, these memory problems and personality changes were significant and very distressing to the family.

- Dealing with the diagnosis openly, taking a problem-oriented approach and providing ongoing practical, psychological and emotional support is much more effective than simply giving a diagnosis.

- Planning for the future. This was one of Mrs R's greatest concerns. Financial and legal information was necessary. Employment and pension issues also had to be negotiated.

- Dealing with these practicalities helped Mr and Mrs R build up a relationship with their CPN and social worker, and begin to come to terms with their situation. Contacts with the local carers group and voluntary organisations were arranged.

- There was a striking contrast between the high stress level in Mrs R and Mr R's apparent lack of concern.

- Early counselling involved beginning the process of helping Mrs R come to terms with the changes in her husband, and in their relationship, at the same time being alert to Mr R's awareness of problems and respond appropriately.

Case study 3: Mr M

Mr M was referred while in hospital for investigation into chronic anaemia (found to be due to low Vitamin B12 and folate levels), 'drop attacks' and cardiac failure. The nursing staff in the ward noticed that he had difficulty in finding the bathroom, could not always find the smoking room and displayed a poor short-term memory in conversation.

Mr M was a 56-year-old gentleman who lived at home with his wife. He was a railway worker who had taken early retirement and his wife still worked as a teacher. They had a son and daughter living nearby, both of whom were married with their own families. He was well supported at home by his wife, who was physically well, and also by the rest of the family, who were in regular contact. Mr M's son-in-law had noticed the memory problems recently, although the rest of the family had some difficulty in accepting or acknowledging them. The initial medical impression was that Mr M had a mild degree of dementia, probably of vascular origin, but his folic acid and B12 deficiency might also be contributing to his mental impairment.

Mr M refused further investigations into his memory problems, his anaemia was treated in hospital and arrangements were made for him to receive further treatment in the community. From the point of view of his memory problems, clinical interview had confirmed the diagnosis of dementia, though the exact cause could not be investigated further. The diagnosis was discussed with his wife, family and also with him. The prognosis in general terms was also discussed, and the need to plan for the future. The family were given regular CPN support via the community mental health team, a social work assessment was completed and appropriate home care was provided to enable Mrs M to continue in her employment.

The couple made wills and enduring Power of Attorney was granted by Mr and Mrs M in favour of their children. Six months later Mrs M developed a chest infection and cough, which would not resolve. Her GP arranged a chest X-ray which demonstrated a large and inoperable lung tumour. Within three days Mrs M had been admitted to hospital for further investigation and treatment.

Sadly Mrs M died within six weeks of her admission to hospital, never having been well enough to return home. By this time Mr M had become considerably more forgetful and was unable to manage his financial affairs. He would have been unable to grant Power of Attorney. Both his family and Mr M were glad that many practical issues surrounding his dementia had been explored and resolved early on in his illness, as this made dealing with the loss of Mrs M and caring for Mr M easier to cope with from a practical point of view.

Issues about diagnosis

The diagnosis of early onset dementing disorders is very inexact, even when patients are assessed in a specialised, multidisciplinary setting (Ferran and Wilson 1996). In a recent paper describing the findings a cohort of people assessed by the specialist early onset services in Liverpool (Ferran and Wilson 1996), almost one-third of the patients could not be given a specific diagnosis after initial assessment, and after a one-year follow up almost one-tenth still had no diagnosis other than 'unspecified dementia'.

This clearly has serious implications for the person with dementia and their partner, as it is more difficult to discuss the likely progression of the disease in anything other than general terms. As there are considerable difficulties in making a correct diagnosis even in specialist settings, and the numbers of people with younger onset dementia in each health authority or health board region are likely to remain relatively small (McGonigal et al. 1993; Newens et al. 1993), it would appear sensible to recommend the development of centres of regional or supra-regional expertise (Health Advisory Service (HAS) 1996). Such centres need to articulate closely with specialists at more local levels, community mental health teams and primary care services. Uncertainties about diagnosis confirm the need to ensure systematic monitoring and review, and the appointment of a case manager or key worker to ensure contact is not lost.

It can be difficult to know how much information to give the person with dementia and their partner or close relatives. The danger is that very limited information or false reassurance can make caring and planning even more stressful. Non-specialist doctors are often shy of giving the diagnosis of dementia; common fears expressed are: 'There's no treatment, so why tell?' or 'It'll be too upsetting for them'.

In practice, most people with younger onset dementia, in the early stages of the disease, know there is something wrong, and are relieved to know the diagnosis. The commonest fears are that they are 'going mad', or have a brain tumour. If giving the diagnosis is handled sensitively and positively, with the assurance of long term support and help, then it is rarely as devastating as the person delivering it imagines.

The issue of insight should also be addressed. Many people have insight into their illness, especially early on, and as the disease progresses, this often declines. Experienced workers suggest that the majority of people have an awareness that their memory for recent events is declining, and that they are becoming more forgetful as time goes on. Some people with dementia are incapable of full insight because of the degree of their dementia, and others may choose to deny insight. It is important to validate the experiences of the person with dementia, and to give an explanation for the often bewildering symptoms which they are experiencing. This is especially important for their partner or close relative, who is often at a loss to understand the changes taking place.

All of this information is far too much to share in one or even two sessions, and needs to be dealt with gradually, in the context of a trusting, supportive relationship, over a period of weeks or months.

It is well known that very few people retain even up to 50 per cent of the content of a consultation, therefore the family should be given the opportunity to discuss their feelings and queries at a later date. It is important that they are given support and counselling throughout this difficult time. They should know that support and help will be ongoing, and that help will be on hand to address both psychological and practical difficulties in the time ahead. The knowledge that there is someone on hand to help with everyday problems, who knows and understands the stresses experienced by both the person with younger onset dementia and the carer, is in itself usually an enormous help. The support of commonly shared experiences in groups such as those run by the Alzheimer's organisations, the Huntington's disease societies, and other groups for specialist conditions can often increase the caring network and decrease the feeling of isolation so often felt (Duff and Peach 1994).

Conclusion

In summary, relatively little research has been carried out on the medical and psychosocial aspects of younger onset dementia in comparison with that of late onset although some of these issues will be addressed later in the book. There is, of course, much common ground in the medical and scientific research into the diseases causing dementia at any age, but the social implications and management are very different. A great deal more research is needed, particularly good-quality, large-scale prevalence and incidence studies across the United Kingdom to assess numbers and needs, and to begin to provide a flexible and responsive service to this group of people.

CHAPTER 2

Epidemiological Issues and Younger People with Dementia

Kirstie Woodburn

Introduction

'The discipline of epidemiology is concerned with the investigation and understanding of factors which relate to the occurrence, natural history and associations of diseases' (Jagger and Lindesay 1993, p.41). The methodology is increasingly being applied to evaluation of service provision and treatment programmes.

This chapter explores some of the methodological problems associated with establishing the extent of early onset dementia, its natural history and possible aetiological factors. Though these issues are relevant to all age groups they are particularly important in the younger age groups where the prevalence (extent) of dementia is relatively low.

In addition, the chapter contains a review of the current literature in this field, and the summary of a recent study in the Lothian area.

Definitions

The extent of a condition in the population can be defined in terms of either incidence or prevalence:

- *incidence* is the proportion of people in a specific population developing a condition over a fixed period of time
- *prevalence* is the number of people in a specific population suffering from a condition at a fixed time.

Early onset or presenile dementia is arbitrarily defined as beginning before the age of 65. It is a much rarer condition than the late onset (senile) form. As yet only a small number of studies have attempted to establish figures for prevalence.

The chapter will attempt to answer the following questions:

1. Why is prevalence and incidence important?
2. What is dementia and who develops it?
3. Why is the stage at which the diagnosis is made so important?
4. Why do different studies give different figures?

In a review of the literature, Liston (1979) states that:

> There are in fact relatively few composite or systematic clinical studies of presenile dementia of even modest sample size; and many of these, it will be seen, present, with the general exception of demographic information, conflicting pictures... Reported epidemiological data, symptoms and signs, and results of ancillary tests often vary widely from study to study, especially as regards findings of history and of mental status and neurological examinations... Indeed on the basis of the literature, one might even question whether there exists a syndrome called presenile dementia, which can be characterised on the clinical grounds with reasonable reliability in the absence of definitive pathological study. (p.329)

Why is prevalence and incidence important?

Epidemiological research enhances the understanding of a particular disease in several ways:

*   accurately determining the prevalence and incidence of a condition enables risk factors to be more accurately identified
*   questions as to whether a condition is becoming more common can only be answered if the figures at the first point in time are known
*   In terms of early onset dementia, such figures can help policy makers and service providers make decisions based on the patterns of the needs they identify.

As emphasised in Chapter 3 on needs assessment, an examination of statistics provides an indication as to how many people might develop early onset dementia in a given locality. This facilitates the provision of comprehensive and adequate health and social care services for them. The definition of need and subsequent delivery of services is equally relevant to relatives and carers. If the results from a local survey are not available the extrapolation of the findings of an appropriate survey elsewhere on the frequency of the condition, would allow some indicative planning so long as account is taken of local demographic characteristics. In areas where the identified target population falls short of the expected total, concerns should be raised as to the adequate detection of the cases. Efforts could then be made to identify such individuals or define other reasons for difference in prevalence.

Service planning is not a particular matter for this chapter, but two key issues which arise and are of immediate relevance to the discussion of the prevalence of the early onset dementia are:

1. The small numbers and geographical spread of the group within one area mean that any 'centralised' service would necessitate the provision of adequate transport facilities to and from it. A better use of resources might therefore be the provision of individualised home-based support.

2. The numbers of new cases being referred over time may affect levels of specialist and non-specialist services.

What is dementia and who develops it?

An important starting point is to look at the definition of dementia and so decide who should be included when a population is studied.

Dementia is used in two contexts which must be clearly distinguished. First, it is used to describe a group of *specific disease entities*; and second, to refer to a *clinical syndrome* which can have a wide range of causes.

When denoting a *syndrome*, the term is best defined as an acquired global impairment of intellect, memory and personality, but without impairment of consciousness. (As such it is almost always of long duration, usually progressive, and often irreversible.)

Certain intrinsic degenerative diseases of the brain occurring in middle or late life have attained the title of dementia as signifying *specific disease entities*. These are the so-called primary dementias, and need to be distinguished from secondary degenerative brain processes. These latter are dementias secondary to the pathological processes underlying them, such as the cerebrovascular disease underlying multi-infarct dementia. (Further information is provided in Chapter 1.)

The next question is, taking the broad definition of dementia, what are the most commonly found causes for the condition? Among the younger onset dementias it is probable that Alzheimer's disease is more frequent than others. This group may in fact be made up of a number of different subtypes of dementia. With the current range of clinical differentiations, division into different subgroups often relates current research interests and prevailing fashions rather than syndromes with important clinical implications. The position, for example, of Lewy Body dementia in the frequency table of dementias needs to be clarified; although McKeith *et al.* (1994), believe that it may represent the second most common form of dementia. Next in frequency could be arteriosclerotic or multi-infarct type dementia. Pick's disease, Huntington's disease and Creutzfeldt-Jakob disease constitute the best-known of the remaining primary dementias and are all very much less common.

An exhaustive list of all the rarer forms of dementia would have to include neurological and medical conditions, such as epilepsy and diabetes, where cognitive decline is only a mild feature of the overall clinical picture. Another example would be HIV-related dementia, but here the overall clinical picture trumps the additional presentation of a dementing illness, in a patient whose survival time is severely shortened. There are consequently a number of specialities which would need to be included if a comprehensive survey of cases were to be made, but few would require services relevant to those with the more common forms.

There obviously is a major challenge in defining what the condition includes, who it affects, and how it should be defined, particularly when it occurs as part of another condition. A specific example is the overlap between multi-infarct dementia and cerebrovascular disease. Though a stroke may contribute to dementia, it is not necessarily the cause. The assessment of cognitive deficiency in cerebrovascular disease is notoriously difficult and it is the presenting symptomatology which decides to which speciality a stroke case is referred. Predominant physical impairments would be the province of physicians in geriatric medicine, general physicians and neurologists, whereas people with cognitive effects would tend to be cared for by the old age psychiatrists and counted as cases of dementia. The overall pattern of impairment would influence whether the patient was specifically diagnosed as having dementia, and entered on a register as such.

Categorisation tends to divide dementia into progressive and non-progressive forms. First, taking the progressive forms of dementia, there are many distinct dementias to include: Alzheimer's, multi-infarct, Pick's, Lewy Body and Parkinson's disease with associated cognitive decline, the extremely rare spongiform encephalopathies such as Creutzfeldt-Jakob disease, and Huntington's disease. There is also the significant problem of Alzheimer's disease occurring in the population of Down's syndrome adults.

The diversity of these disorders raises the obvious difficulty for service providers in meeting the needs of such a range within a single service.

Non-progressive categories of dementia share many of the problems with progressive forms. Cases of post head-injured patients displaying behavioural problems and cognitive deficiencies are one such example.

The differential diagnosis of a primary degenerative younger onset dementia is very extensive, ranging from a depressive illness to a space-occupying lesion (see Figure 2.1).

Degenerative: Alzheimer's disease, Pick's disease and other frontal dementias, Huntington's chorea, Parkinson's disease, Creutzfeldt-Jakob disease, normal pressure hydrocephalus, multiple sclerosis.

Intracranial space – occupying lesions: tumour, subdural haematoma.

Traumatic: single severe head injuries, repeated head injuries in boxers etc.

Infections and related conditions: encephalitis of any cause, neurosyphilis, cerebral sarcoidosis, HIV, prion diseases.

Vascular: vascular dementia including multi-infarct, occlusion of the carotid artery, cranial arthritis, systemic lupus erythematosis.

Metabolic: sustained uraemia, liver failure, remote effects of carcinoma or lymphoma, renal dialysis, diabetes mellitus. (There may be a mild degree of impairment in many cases. This can be much more severe in patients who have suffered multiple episodes of hypoglycaemia.)

Toxic: alcohol, poisoning with heavy metals such as: lead, arsenic, thallium.

Drugs: benzodiapines, phenothiazines, tricyclic antidepressants, digoxin, cimetidene.

Anoxia: anaemia, post-anaesthesia, carbon monoxide, cardiac arrest, chronic respiratory failure.

Vitamin lack: sustained lack of B12, folic acid, thiamine, nicotinic acid.

Pseudodementia: alcohol and drug dependence, physical illness, functional psychiatric disorder: depression, hypomania/mania, schizophrenia, hysteria.

Other organic psychosyndromes: Korsakoff psychosis, drug toxicity, delirium, epilepsy.

Figure 2.1 Causes of dementia (adapted from the *Oxford Textbook of Psychiatry,* Gelder *et al.* 1996, p.314)

Diagnostic criteria

The standard clinical diagnostic criteria for dementia are briefly described in the International Classification of Diseases, 10th edition, ICD-10 (World Health Organisation 1992) and the Diagnostic and Statistical Manual 4th edition, DSM-IV (American Psychiatric Association, 1994), the two main diagnostic systems. These allow some distinction between the different types of the condition. Figure 2.2 gives DSM-IV criteria for Alzheimer's dementia. Other criteria aim to provide more reliable clinical diagnoses during life, such as the McKhann criteria for Alzheimer's type dementia (McKhann *et al.* 1984) and others for vascular dementia (Chui *et al.* 1992; Roman *et al.* 1993). Attempts are currently being made to develop internationally agreed criteria for Lewy Body dementia also.

It is important to stress that the most reliable way to establish a diagnosis is to perform a neuropathological examination after death. Even this some-times can generate confusion when several pathologies coexist. Perhaps as our molecular and genetic understanding of these illnesses increase and brain scanning techniques become even more sophisticated, it will be possible to define dementias with great accuracy and during the lifetime of the person. This may indeed run in parallel with the development of novel forms of treat-ment related to a more effective grasp of changes in the molecular biology of these conditions.

Why is the stage at which diagnosis is made so important?

Another factor which influences measurement of the size of the problem in a population is its recognition. In other words, there should be information on when it is possible to make a diagnosis and how straightforward this is. Rele-vant and related issues are the mechanism and routes of referral for diagnosis and assessment.

Regrettably the diagnosis of early onset dementia is problematic, espe-cially in its early stages. This interferes with the epidemiological analysis and, far more significantly, can greatly add to the difficulties and distress of the person involved and their relatives. Diagnostic problems inevitably cause delays: both in people with dementia asking for help and in health profes-sionals identifying the presenting features as early onset dementia.

The family may initially explain away the onset and progress of very insidious and worrying symptoms as stress-related or they may attempt to 'cover-up' and deny that there are difficulties. This makes it notoriously diffi-cult to establish when the onset of the illness took place. There may thus be a considerable time between the presentation of symptoms and establishing a 'hospital diagnosis'. The latter may well be the most accurate point in time available. One way in which this causes an underestimate of early onset cases is that if symptoms begin at age 64 but the diagnosis is made at 66, this case will be misclassified.

Even if relatives recognise and accept that there are difficulties for the person and themselves coping, the next problem is access to and involvement of the family doctor. An example is that someone with the cognitive impairments may be very unwilling to see the doctor, denying the deficit, or feeling threatened by such a suggestion. Further delay ensues; further tension and worry accumulate.

The progressive nature of the condition means that, in addition to mental health problems, disturbed relationships within the family and behavioural problems may follow, leading to increased levels of stress so that contact with the GP is almost inevitable at some stage of the illness. When eventually the GP is made aware of the issues, it is more than likely that he or she will refer to a specialist for diagnostic assessment. This is more likely in younger people where the unexpected nature of cognitive decline in youth or middle age makes looking for treatable causes, such as tumour and so on, particularly relevant and urgent.

Involvement of other relevant health and social care professionals would partly depend on the local service organisation and its coordination, but also on the particular problem presented. This could result in either a neurological or psychiatric referral. For example, neurological symptoms might lead to a neurological referral, while predominant behaviour problems would be considered to be within the realm of a psychiatrist. Referral to a specialist centre or memory clinic would be more likely if the GP sought a multidisciplinary assessment.

Even with the aid of brain scanning equipment, the diagnoses of certain forms of dementia are only made by excluding other possible causes. In less clear-cut cases, the use of serial assessments or reviews to document cognitive decline is often the best approach, rather than categorising the condition from the scant information gleaned from one visit to a specialist. An inevitable consequence is that there is further delay before there can be reasonable certainty about the diagnosis.

The difficulties of making early diagnoses are also illustrated in two studies of sufferers from early onset dementia seen in psychiatric settings. In one of these, follow-up of patients diagnosed as having early onset dementia revealed a high prevalence of wrong diagnoses (Ron *et al.* 1979). Out of 52 cases, 51 were followed up between 5 and 15 years on and the initial diagnosis was rejected in 16. Nott and Fleminger (1975) followed up 35 patients diagnosed as having early onset dementia and in only 15 cases did progressive deterioration confirm the diagnosis. The issue of differential diagnosis and outcome of early onset dementia has also been studied in samples of neuropsychiatric referrals (Freemon 1976; Victoratos, Lenman and Herzberg 1977; Marsden and Harrison 1972; Smith and Kiloh 1981). Subjects in the samples had a variety of ages but generally had early onset. Such studies further emphasised the importance of investigation for reversible causes of dementia in younger age groups.

Such surveys from neurological units have reported on the evaluation of in-patients consecutively admitted to hospital with a presumptive diagnosis of dementia. Since the majority of the patients were below the age of 65, the results can be seen as an indication of what could be expected in an early onset group. The most important observation is that about 15 per cent, after full evaluation, were not thought to be suffering from dementia but to have some other organic psychosyndrome or functional psychiatric disorder.

A study of 200 patients under the age of 65 by Ferran *et al.* (1996) also point to problems and complexity of diagnosis. The authors conclude that there is a need for multidisciplinary services for this group of people.

The prevalence of a condition is related to the frequency with which the condition occurs, length of time that sufferers survive and the ability to successfully detect cases. As previously indicated, the definition of onset can be at the age of symptom onset or the age of diagnosis; and the latter is probably the more reliable of the two. This clearly affects the comparison of age-specific rates when based on age at onset. The progress of the illness, its duration and overall survival time will likewise be influenced by this. Dealing with a heterogeneous condition means that differences between subgroups may get lost in overall figures.

In calculating prevalence, an appropriate age range must also be chosen. The rather arbitrary cut-off point usually taken is 65 years, but at what lower end should a line be drawn? This is commonly the age of 40 or 45 years and it is reasonable to assume that an age onset after 30 years will effectively exclude all cases of learning disability.

The essential for establishing a prevalence figure is that there should be an accurate estimate for the population for the age range in question and that the time period should be clearly specified during which the cases were identified.

Why do different studies give different figures?

As the previously quoted extract from Liston indicates, studies in the current literature often give conflicting results for prevalence. Is there an explanation for this inconsistency?

It can be explained by asking questions about how cases were ascertained and by scrutinising details of the methodology in each study. In estimating the prevalence of early onset dementia, how extensive has the search been, how have cases been defined, and what have the inclusion and exclusion criteria been?

Some health services have computerised patient registers which facilitates the identification of cases with a specified diagnosis. However, these systems are prone to error related to factors such as inaccurate data, duplication of the same case, misclassification and miscoding. Other research groups have looked at case note information, and depended for their diagnoses on the clinical information provided by these rather than on live individual assessments.

Other pertinent questions are as follows.

- Have all potential parts of the service been explored? For example, psychiatric (general adult psychiatric and psychiatry of old age), neurological and medical sources, as well as old age physicians.
- Have in-patient, out-patient (including memory clinics) and day hospitals been included?
- What of community contacts such as nursing homes, both private and public, and day centres?

As has already been indicated, the majority of cases would be likely to be referred to these services. A very small number of people could theoretically be missed – say, if they were living rough and not registered with a GP, or if the dementia was associated with such concomitant problems (e.g. heavy alcohol abuse) as to make assessment of underlying cognitive decline very difficult.

It is clear that such surveys result in a loss of cases due to missing notes unmet criteria and so on. Further attrition occurs in studies involving the contact of cases due to events such as death, migration from the area, or simply because an individual or his/her carers refuse to participate.

Some previous prevalence studies have used data collected from populations of all ages within which are a substantial proportion of cases below the age of 65 years. None of these has been UK-based. There are only a few studies concentrating on younger onset cases and the number of cases in these is usually small so that there are correspondingly large confidence intervals. Comparison is also bedevilled by the use of different case-finding techniques. An exception is that prevalence rates for presenile dementia of the Alzheimer's type (PDAT) are consistent across several studies. This must be due to well-defined criteria being used to make the diagnosis.

A further point is that only some studies were based on population sampling and individual assessment and these are probably biased towards the more severe forms of the conditions.

One of the most important attempts to consolidate information on the prevalence of dementia of all ages was the European Concerted Action on the Epidemiology and Prevention of Dementia study (EURODEM). This looked at 12 prevalence studies of dementia conducted in eight European countries between 1980 and 1990 (Hofman *et al.* 1991). Following reanalysis of the original data they produced the overall prevalence estimates shown in Table 2.1.

Table 2.1 EURODEM Prevalence rate (percentage of total population) of dementia by age group and gender

Age group	Both sexes	Women	Men
30–59	0.1	0.1	0.2
60–64	1.0	0.5	1.6
65–69	1.4	1.1	2.2
70–74	4.1	3.9	4.6
75–79	5.7	6.7	5.0
80–84	13.0	13.5	12.1
85–89	21.6	22.8	18.5
90–94	32.2	32.2	32.1
95–99	34.7	36.0	31.6

Source: Adapted from Hofman *et al.* 1991

This table usefully provides prevalence rates according to gender and age group. Subjects included in the reanalysis were all assessed using DSM-III or equivalent and individual examination; institutionalised populations were included in the samples.

In a Finnish urban study (Molsa, Marttila and Rinne 1982) the diagnosis of dementia was supported by neurological testing and laboratory investigations, and used hospital data and reports from community agencies. The prevalence figure for degenerative dementia, for 45–64-year-olds, was 46.7/100,000 (17 cases in a population of 36,409).

In the Finnish national study, Sulkava *et al.* (1985) used personal interviews and psychological tests to make a diagnosis and based rates on a probability sample from the general adult population. Their figure for primary degenerative dementia, for 30–64-year-olds, was 32.7/100,000 (2 cases in a population of 6,120).

In Copiah County, Mississippi, Schoenberg, Anderson and Haerer (1985) used interviews and neurological examinations to detect dementia, and included all households and institutions. For 40–64-year-olds, the figures for PDAT were 18.2/100,000 (1 case in a population of 5,489). In their 1987 figure, the calculated incidence for probable presenile Alzheimer's disease was 2.4/100,000.

In the Rochester (USA) study, Kokmen *et al.* (1989) used a system of ascertainment incorporating general practice records and nursing homes, and described as 'centralised medical record-linkage system'. The group's 1988 figure for PDAT, for 45–64-year-olds, was 31.8/100,000 (3 cases in a population of 9,431).

A study of the incidence of early onset dementia was based on the Israeli National Neurological Disease Register, and the clinical records of all patients between the ages of 43 and 60 years discharged in Israel between 1974 and 1983 with a neurological or psychiatric diagnosis suggesting dementia (Treves *et al.* 1986). Individuals entering institutions were identified, and the date of onset of the condition established by interviewing informants retrospectively. This gave an incidence of 2.4/100,000/year for individuals aged 40 to 60 years.

In 1993, McGonigal *et al.* did a retrospective review of all hospital records in Scotland (of patients less than 75 years old with various diagnoses of dementia) who had been admitted to psychiatric hospitals, as well as from neurology out-patients and general hospitals. This was to ascertain the cases of PDAT between 1974 and 1988, with an onset between 40 and 64 years.

This gave an annual incidence of probable Alzheimer's disease of 1.6. The incidence, between the ages of 40 and 64, was 22.6/100,000 for probable Alzheimer's disease. Denominators for incidence were taken from the 1981 census. The paper was criticised as its rates were based predominantly on admission to psychiatric hospitals. There also was concern about its claim that there was an increased risk to women. It also used a classification for multi-infarct dementia based on the Hachinski score which did not take into account the group of mixed aetiology (Hachinski *et al.* 1975).

Newens *et al.* (1993), published figures for clinically diagnosed PDAT, under 65 years, in the Northern Health Region, England, for the years 1979–1986. This was based on the case ascertainment through medical and other care agencies, by case note review. They argue that prevalence would be 25 per cent underestimated if in-patient data alone were used, rather than their system of day hospital, and neuroradiology records being included as well. From the same source, Newens goes on to say: 'The assessment of true need requires therefore that data are collated from a variety of health, social and voluntary sources, underlining the importance of completeness and accuracy in health information systems' (Newens *et al.* 1993, p.643).

The data did not suggest that PDAT runs an especially malignant course and has a shorter survival than older groups, and so does not support age-related heterogeneity in this way. The prevalence per 100,000 of different types of dementia for the Northern Health Region, for people 45–64 years was:

Alzheimer's (PDAT)   = 34.6 (227 cases, population = 655,800).

Vascular   = 11.7

Other (secondary)   = 27.0

Total   = 73.3

The point prevalence was estimated at 34.6/100,000.

The annual incidence of dementia was 3.4/100,000 for those aged 40–60 years, rising to 7.2/100,000 for those aged 45–64 years.

The pattern was of diagnosis followed by a period in community care. It was estimated that for an average health district with a population of 60,000, between the ages of 45 and 64, about 20 people would be identified with PDAT and that more than 50 per cent of them would require hospital or community support for over five years.

A. The development of multiple cognitive deficits manifested by both:

    (1) memory impairment (impaired ability to learn new information or to recall previously learned information)

    (2) one (or more) of the following cognitive disturbances:

        (a) aphasia (language disturbance)

        (b) apraxia (impaired ability to carry out motor activities despite intact motor function)

        (c) agnosia (failure to recognise or identify objects despite intact sensory function)

        (d) disturbance in executive functioning (i.e. planning, organising, sequencing, abstracting).

B. The cognitive deficits in Criteria A1 and A2 each cause significant impairment in social or occupational functioning and represent a significant decline from a previous level of functioning.

C. The course is characterised by gradual onset and continuing cognitive decline.

D. The cognitive deficits in Criteria A1 and A2 are not due to any of the following:

    (1) other central nervous system conditions that cause progressive deficits in memory and cognition (e.g. cerebrovascular disease, Parkinson's disease, Huntington's disease, subdural haematoma, normal pressure hydrocephalus, brain tumour)

    (2) systemic conditions that are known to cause dementia (e.g, hypothroidism, vitamin B12 or folic acid deficiency, niacin deficiency, hypercalcemia, neurosyphilis, HIV infection)

    (3) substance-induced conditions.

E. The deficits do not occur exclusively during the course of a delirium.

F. The disturbance is not better accounted for by another Axis disorder (e.g. major depressive disorder, schizophrenia).

Figure 2.2 DSM-IV criteria for dementia of the Alzheimer's type *(American Psychiatric Association 1994)*

A bulletin from the Royal College of Psychiatrists (Ferran and Wilson 1997) produced the following estimates:

> Recent epidemiological studies have yielded conflicting results, but we can tentatively assume that a consultant responsible for the care of people with dementia should have to expect, in an average district of 200,000 inhabitants younger than 65, between 14 and 45 new cases of Alzheimer's Disease plus 40 new cases of Multi-infarct Dementia. An average of two new referrals every week should be expected if all were referred to the service.

An example

The following is an illustrated example of the investigation of early onset dementia, taken from research on the clinical profiles, patterns of decline and genetic information of patients with early onset dementia in Lothian area, Scotland, by Dr K Woodburn and Professor E Johnstone of the Department of Psychiatry, University of Edinburgh.

Background

The study aim was to identify a population of live patients in the Lothian area of Scotland, with early onset dementia of various aetiologies, to describe the clinical profiles of each person and the patterns of decline which occur, together with any genetic information.

Methods

Cases of early onset dementia were identified using the Lothian Psychiatric Case Register. All subjects were assessed by the one clinician. For demographic data, the CAMDEX (The Cambridge Examination for Mental Disorders of the Elderly) informant interview was used. Behavioural assessment was based on the CAPE-BRS (Clifton Assessment Procedure for the Elderly, Behavioural Rating Scale), the Cornell Depression Scale and the MOUSEPAD (Manchester and Oxford University scale for the Psychopathological Assessment of Dementia), a new behavioural and psychopathological assessment. Where possible the *cognitive assessment* was completed using the NART (National Adult Reading Test) and CAMCOG (cognitive assessment of the CAMDEX). A physical and neurological examination was done and the Webster scale for Parkinsonian features included. Forty millilitres of blood was taken for the genetic analysis at the assessment interview. After an interval of approximately one year, each case was reassessed using these instruments.

Results

Of 290 potential cases of dementia identified, 164 (57%) were excluded (for reasons including death, wrong diagnosis, refusal, untraceability). Of the 126 (43%) cases seen, there were 53 (42%) male, 73 (58%) female, with an average age at original referral of 58 years.

A total of 114 cases met the *Diagnostic and Statistical Manual of Mental Disorders*, (American Psychiatric Association 1987) criteria for dementia: 60 (52%) for Alzheimer's type dementia; 13 (11%) for multi-infarct dementia; 14 (12%) for alcohol-related dementia, with 25 (22%) in a mixed group overlapping these categories; and 2 (1%) in other dementia types.

A full description of the group and the results of follow up, together with the genetic characterisation, is available from the author.

Important data concerning the services provided and used by this group of patients and their carers has been collected and can be shared with organisations working to make the case for funding for early onset dementia in the health and social services.

Conclusions

This study provides a thoroughly documented and clinically detailed sample. The analysis of the work may help to identify if subgroups exist, according to the patterns of various clinical features, the rates of decline, and genetic variations. This will in turn, give a greater chance to plan appropriately for all those involved in caring for and managing these illnesses.

Acknowledgement

With grateful thanks to Emeritus Professor W. MacLennan for his help in revising the draft of this chapter and to the Wellcome Trust for their research grant to perform the above study.

CHAPTER 3

Needs Assessment
Individual and Strategic Care Planning
Gregor McWalter and James Chalmers

Introduction

The popularity of the term 'needs assessment' has boomed since the introduction of the community care reforms heralded in the White Paper *Caring
for People* (Department of Health 1989). The term is used widely in both
health and social care, and may refer to a number of concepts underpinning
the relationship between service providers and users.

'Needs assessment' is used widely in the practical application of
assessment as an activity of care. At the time of the community care reforms,
and subsequently, such applications have been widely encouraged for both
practitioners (e.g. Smale *et al.* 1993; Social Services Inspectorate (SSI) 1991a)
and managers (e.g. SSI 1991b). The wide use of the term is reflected in early
and continuing discussion and debate in the literature. Such discussion
continues (e.g. Nolan and Caldock 1995; McWalter 1997), in part because
the applications and meanings of the term 'needs assessment' are wide and
often diffuse (Nolan and Caldock 1995; McWalter *et al.* 1994).

While the debates continue over needs assessment as an activity which
underpins individual care, there is a further application of the term which
refers to the assessment of need in populations. It may be argued that this
application originated in the rise of population medicine – although clearly it
is equally important in social care.

However, the meaning and application of the term is diffuse. This is in
part through necessity and quite appropriate – the assessment of population
needs by its nature requires a range of techniques.

Thus the term 'needs assessment' may be used to refer to the assessment of
the needs of either individuals or populations. In either context the precise

definition and application of the term, conceptually and in implementation, may vary between agencies, professions and individuals. This chapter will focus on these two distinct but related aspects of needs assessment: the assessment of individuals and that of populations.

To meet the needs of younger people with dementia, in both individuals and the population, good needs assessment is vital. The needs of this group are likely to differ from that of older people with dementia, for example in the importance of employment or perhaps of dependent children, yet knowledge of the needs and what is required to address them is still being developed (e.g. Cox and McLennan 1994). Given the tendency of practitioners to think in terms of what services are available, rather than needs (DoH 1993), and that specialised services for younger people with dementia are rare, accurate information about needs is central to both service delivery on an individual basis and for the planning and development of services.

Individual need

In emphasising the importance of needs assessment in delivering high-quality care, the community care reforms clearly prescribed a change in the working practice of many practitioners in both health and social care. Such a change was often welcomed – one indicator of this is the local development of 'needs assessment tools' in both health and social care agencies, although particularly in the latter given their statutory obligations. However, while much of the literature pertaining to the community care reforms did specify what information should be collected in a needs assessment (e.g. Centre for Policy on Ageing 1990; SSI 1991a) there was less emphasis on what 'need' actually meant. Where definition was attempted (e.g. SSI 1991a) it often served to illustrate the difficulty of the task, for example employing concepts such as dependency and quality of life, themselves subject to problems of definition (McWalter et al. 1994).

While definitions have been proposed (e.g. McWalter et al. 1994), the debate over the definition of need and its implications for the practice of needs assessment continues (e.g. Nolan and Caldock 1995). However, clear definition is important for the assessment of individual need. Community care often requires complex multidisciplinary working and this is particularly true for the care required by people with dementia. Such cooperation between professions and agencies is vital for seamless care, and depends in part on a shared understanding of common concepts for effective communication and understanding (McWalter et al. 1994). While confusion over what constitutes 'need' remains, effective multidisciplinary working may be compromised, for example particularly where health and social care providers are approaching the provision of care from potentially different perspectives. In addition, where joint working requires the development, evaluation and application of shared assessment tools, a common and clearly stated definition of need is required. The reliability and validity of such tools as assessments of need will depend on such a definition. In particular, validity as an evaluative criteria (e.g. Peck and Shapiro 1990) cannot be established in the absence of a clear definition of the concept which the tool purports to measure.

A clarification within the concept of need concerns the distinction between an identified difficulty and the help required to address it. Such a distinction applies at both an individual (Thayer 1973) and population level (Stewart 1979) and entails a number of implications (McWalter *et al.* 1994), for example that dependency and disability do not necessarily predict either the type or extent of met or unmet need. The difficulties which an individual may experience become indicators of potential need; they may or may not constitute unmet need depending on the individual's current circumstances in terms of individual strengths, support networks and preferences.

It is unmet need which is usually the subject of assessment for health and social care, albeit usually implicitly. However, the assessment of how current needs are met is important for supplying information about the strengths of service users and carers, and about personal and social networks (e.g. Wilcox, Jones and Alldrick 1995).

The assessment of an individual's difficulties are vital in a needs assessment; such difficulties engender need. However, a needs assessment must also assess what is required to address those difficulties and do so in terms independent of existing services. This is in line with the spirit and letter of the community care reforms outlined in *Caring for People* (DoH 1989) – the assessment of need should not rely on current service provision.

Assessing and recording the help required to address difficulties in individual assessments may be achieved by employing the notion of 'types of help' (McWalter *et al.* 1994). These comprise a specification of need in terms of the caring activities required to address the needs engendered by specific problems, for example a person with dementia who had an unmet need with bathing might require one or more of the following: bathing aids, prompting with bathing or physical assistance with bathing, depending on their current preferences and support. These caring activities are independent of the actual service provision, and often of the profession or sector (e.g. health or social care) which should provide the help (although this is implicit in some types of help for particular problems, for example a need for 'specialist assessment' for problems with 'physical health' implies intervention from a medical practitioner). The notion of types of help offers one solution to the problem that practitioners may tend to think in terms of services (DoH 1993).

The foregoing suggests that the assessment of need is distinct from assessing other aspects of a person, for example either total or excess disability, dependency or mental state. This conflicts with descriptions of many current assessment tools as 'needs assessments', for example behaviour and dependency ratings (e.g. Revised Elderly Person's Disability Scale; Fleming and Bowles 1994; Clifton Assessment Procedure for the Elderly; Pattie and Gilleard 1979), mental status examinations (e.g. Mini-Mental State Examination; Folstein, Folstein and McHugh 1975) and indices of carer stress or burden (e.g. the Relative Stress Scale; Greene *et al.* 1982). Such assessments focus on the difficulties which an individual faces and while their role is likely to be vital in some circumstances, they do not assess what is required to address those difficulties. It is possible to incorporate an assessment of types of help into an assessment pro forma, for example the Care Needs Assessment Pack for Dementia (CarenapD) (McWalter *et al.* 1998).

Definitions of need

In considering a definition of need, Bradshaw (1972) proposed a taxonomy of need necessary to account for different types of need, suggesting that there was no single definition. This taxonomy comprises normative need (defined by care professional), perceived need (defined by user), expressed need (perceived need turned into action) and comparative need (in relation to similar populations). Normative and perceived need are of particular relevance to the assessment of individual need. While Bradshaw's taxonomy is not without problems, it is clearly useful as a conceptual tool and as a demonstration of the lack of a single global definition.

Thus need may be defined in the context of the assessment of individual need as 'a state where help...is seen to be required by the care professional making the assessment, taking into account the views of the person assessed or of their advocate' (McWalter *et al.* 1994, p.217). Such a definition applies to the assessment of both the needs of people with dementia and the needs of carers in their own right. In addition, a carer may act as an advocate for a person with dementia. It is vital to note that while the assessment of an individual by a care professional constitutes an application of a normative definition of need, it must also include a recognition and recording of perceived need. In this it attempts to account for potential disagreements between the assessor and the person assessed, for example where a person may not perceive difficulties which the assessor feels are clearly evident, such as with home security or nutrition. Clearly this is a difficult area which underlines the necessity for training, experience, sensitivity and an awareness of personal and cultural values on the part of practitioners assessing people with dementia. Such issues are discussed in the literature (e.g. McWalter 1997; Nolan and Caldock 1995; Smale *et al.* 1993).

It is a criticism of existing assessment tools that they constitute a purely normative approach to assessment, and this is particularly true for measures of dependency and disability. However, it is important to distinguish between assessment tools and a holistic assessment conducted by an experienced practitioner. An assessment tool can never replace the assessment of a skilled practitioner, rather it is best regarded as an aid to assessment which complements the range of skills and techniques which may be included in such an assessment. Individual tools may assess need, dependency or cognitive impairment; it is the choice of the practitioner to apply these tools as appropriate for any individual and to make the best use of the information subsequently recorded.

One aspect of assessment often neglected, particularly for people with dementia, is the voice of the user (e.g. Goldsmith 1996). This might include addressing life history, biographical approaches, family and social networks and current and previous roles and responsibilities. This aspect of assessment would include recording perceived need, but would also assess and record preferences and requirements of the person as they see them. It is recognised that these may conflict with the view of the assessor or carer but no simple solutions are available or appropriate for such conflicts, rather they must be tackled on an individual basis. However, such questions may throw into sharp relief questions regarding the nature of assessment itself.

Carers

The role of carers has in recent years been increasingly recognised as vital. This is often particularly true for community care, and for the care of people with dementia. However, the needs of carers may become subsumed or even lost in considerations of the needs of the person or persons for whom they care. While there are a range of assessment pro formas for many of the disease conditions or client groups requiring care in the community, there are relatively few for carers. In addition, the needs of carers and those for whom they care may conflict, a fact which highlights the need for skilled practice.

Individual needs assessment

In the practice of both health and social care in the community the empowerment of the service user *should* be central in the processes of assessment, care planning and service delivery. In practice, however, such empowerment may be difficult to achieve, despite the best of intentions. Within assessment, the empowerment of the user may be adversely affected by a lack of attention to the voice of the user, a particular problem for people with dementia. Such clients will experience cognitive impairment which make expression and communication difficult. The availability of encouragement and practical techniques for practitioners to address such difficulties is a relatively recent development.

In addition, the development of models of assessment (e.g. Smale *et al.* 1993) and the consequent establishment of principles of good assessment, such as that 'a good assessor will: (1) empower both the user and carer... (2) involve, rather than just inform, the user and carer...be interested in the user and carer as people' (Nolan and Caldock 1995, p.82), are helpful in addressing issues of empowerment. They begin to equip practitioners with the knowledge and skills to conduct the process of assessment in a manner which is empowering to users. Skills essential to the process of assessment include relationship building, ensuring a good environment, avoiding value judgements, keeping an open mind and being interested in the service user and carer as people (Nolan and Caldock 1995). However, it is important to recognise that assessment comprises both process and task.

At its most basic, the task of assessment is to inform, to provide accurate information upon which decisions may be based (McWalter 1997). Yet gathering accurate information may itself be fraught with difficulties. People with dementia may not be aware of their disease or of the difficulties which it causes them. Thus to gather accurate information may require a range of strategies on the part of the assessor, including direct observation or talking to both formal and informal carers. In short, it is in the task of assessment where the advantages of the normative approach to assessment and the application of assessment tools may prove beneficial. However, the empowerment of the user remains central, and can be conceptualised as a thread which runs not only through the process of assessment, but also through care planning and service delivery.

The foregoing helps to illuminate the role of assessment tools in individual assessment – as aids to the task of gathering information within the holistic assessment of the skilled practitioner. It is important to note that the minimum requirements of any assessment tool are that it is both reliable, i.e. consistent between practitioners and through time, and valid, i.e. it assesses what it purports to. The application of appropriate assessment tools aids formal assessments by supplying accurate information about specific aspects of a person, such as need, dependency, functional ability or cognitive impairment.

The individual as part of the population

Many agencies have adopted assessment tools as routine for particular workers or groups of clients. This is particularly true for local authorities, given their statutory responsibilities. The routine application of an appropriate assessment tool by an agency or within a locality represents more than simply a collection of individual assessments. It is through aggregation of such assessments that the process of individual assessment can contribute to the process of assessing the needs of populations. This represents one approach to population needs assessment, termed 'bottom-up'. It contrasts with more traditional, 'top-down' approaches.

Population needs assessment

One of the main intentions of the NHS and community care reforms was the separation of the function of commissioning care from that of delivery. Commissioners of health care such as health authorities (health boards in Scotland) and fundholding GPs are explicitly required to assess the health needs of their resident populations, then address these needs by commissioning services from any suitable provider, after agreeing costs and quality standards. While social services departments have not experienced the same split between commissioners and providers, similar arrangements pertain for assessing the needs of populations. Since 1990 the role of social service departments has changed from providing services for presented need to include a joint (with other health and social care providers), strategic understanding of the population's need for community care (Social Work Services Inspectorate for Scotland (SWSI) 1996).

The deceptively simple concept of 'population needs assessment' was soon found to be fraught with problems – even the definition of 'need' itself was hotly debated (e.g. Stevens and Raftery 1994). Eventually, most organisations commissioning health services accepted that 'need' encompassed an 'ability to benefit', however it remained unclear what this might mean when applied to populations (Kelly *et al.* 1996; Stevens and Raftery 1994). Other difficult questions surfaced, for example whether health care commissioners should aim for the maximum total achievable 'health gain' at the expense of an equitable distribution of resources or whether scarce resources should be given to the sickest members of society, even if their chances of benefiting were small. In addition, it was not clear how investment in prevention should be balanced against expenditure on treatment and care (Williams 1989). A range of similar issues vex social service departments.

At a more practical level, commissioners of health care and planners of social care were faced with having to somehow ensure that all the potential needs of a population were recognised and quantified so that they could be explicitly addressed with appropriate contracts. To contact each individual in a population would be impossible, and even to target those likely to have special health needs would be difficult and time consuming. Ways had to be found to paint a 'broad brush' picture of a population's health needs. The simplest way to provide comprehensive health and social care for a population was to purchase the same services as in previous years, but this stopgap measure was exactly what the reforms were intended to replace. Nevertheless, one of the major influences on the commissioning of any type of care is its historical provision, for example where there has always been extensive psychiatric in-patient provision this is likely to remain more accessible for that local population.

Most commissioners of health care have performed some sort of global screening of health needs within their populations, and then concentrated on areas which are identified to be of particular importance; either because they are common (e.g. heart disease), debilitating (e.g. cancer), treatable (e.g. cataract), expensive (e.g. coronary artery bypass surgery) or perceived to be of considerable importance to society (e.g. drug misuse). In addition, there are a range of other factors which may lead to different diseases being prioritised, for example the activities of pressure groups, the attentions of the media, the advent of new treatments and changing cultural and societal values. Specific features of a needs assessment for younger people with dementia which may make such an assessment difficult are discussed below. Given the increased importance attached to population needs assessment in recent years (SWSI 1996), the approach of social services departments tends to be becoming more similar in many ways to that of commissioners of health care, with the exception of a focus on 'client groups' such as older people or people with learning disabilities rather than specific diseases (although these may coincide in some cases such as dementia or HIV/AIDS).

Features of a population needs assessment

Fundamental to any population needs assessment is an assessment of the incidence and prevalence of the particular condition in question (McEwen, Russell and Stewart 1995), or some sort of 'scoping' of the size of the problem in terms of numbers of people likely to require intervention. This is a relatively straightforward exercise for many 'acute' health conditions, for example the need for services relating to acute myocardial infarction, and some conditions requiring social care, for example people with HIV/AIDS. Given resource constraints, this must be coupled to a scrutiny of the evidence on capacity to benefit, leading to an economic evaluation of the costs and benefits of providing the different possible patterns of care (McEwen *et al.* 1995). For any given area of interest, this top-down approach should in theory give similar answers to a bottom-up approach based on amalgamating the specific needs of all the identified individuals with a specific condition.

In practice, the two approaches are more intertwined. The bottom-up approach requires some sort of population overview to identify the relevant individuals for further scrutiny, and the top-down approach is usually based on data which at some stage are derived from individuals. Also, where routine information is not available, bespoke surveys have to be arranged. These may be based on a random sample, or comprehensive within a geographical area. Such comprehensive studies are in themselves a bottom-up approach, yet the information derived from them may be applied to different populations in a top-down approach. A number of such studies have been conducted for people with dementia (e.g. Gordon and Spicker 1997) and their carers (e.g. Philp *et al.* 1995).

Clearly an estimate of the numbers of people in a population who may require health or social care is not the only issue in population needs assessment, nor in commissioning. It is, however, fundamental.

The Scottish Needs Assessment Programme (SNAP) approach

The Scottish Needs Assessment Programme (McEwen *et al.* 1995) is a health service initiative conceived in response to the realisation that much of the needs assessment work was common to all the health commissioning authorities in Scotland, and that much of the work involved making decisions on the fairest distribution of scarce resources. The Scottish Public Health Forum, a committee set up by the Chief Medical Officer for Scotland, undertook to arrange an alliance of interested bodies to coordinate needs assessment work, and produce a series of comprehensive reports of a standard pattern, relevant to particular facets of health care (Scottish Office 1997b).

Similar reports are produced in England and Wales by the district health authorities (DOHA) project. These reports tend to be more targeted to an epidemiological assessment of the particular areas of need, whereas the SNAP reports include more health economics and greater detail of existing services and their variation across Scotland (McEwen *et al.* 1995). This partly reflects the smaller size of the country, and also the greater sophistication of the available routine health information in Scotland.

Population needs assessment for younger people with dementia

The top-down approach of population needs assessment causes particular problems when applied to the field of younger people with dementia, many of which apply to dementia generally.

Status of younger people with dementia

The resources of population needs assessment tend to be targeted at services which are either expensive, involve many people, or have a particularly high profile. This latter element is a feature of conditions with a high mortality and/or a requirement for expensive hospital care, such as cancer. Unfortunately, dementia in general, and in younger people in particular, is unlikely to figure high on a health commissioning authority's list of areas needing urgent needs assessment, perhaps in part because many people still live at home. However, dementia may now have greater priority, perhaps in part because other more high-profile problems are being gradually understood and addressed. It is also relevant that dementia, and dementia in people under 65 years of age, is a feature of other conditions such as HIV infection, which traditionally seem to have a greater priority, perhaps in part because of a variety of cultural and societal values. The effect of such values are not confined to the health sector, for example social service departments are likely to prioritise child care through values enshrined in part through legislation.

The profile of younger people with dementia may be considerably enhanced if the variant form of Creutzfeldt-Jakob disease takes hold as some authorities fear. Similarly, an increase in the number of people with HIV/AIDS, and the possibility of dementia-related brain impairment, may be important in the future. In addition, the availability of new drug treatments which are likely to prove expensive may also enhance the profile of dementia generally.

Potential for health gain

Areas with a significant potential for health gain as a result of health service intervention are seen as a high priority for needs assessment work. This potential obviously depends on how health gain is measured. Understandably, treatable conditions with an avoidable mortality are seen as having a high potential for health gain. Conditions in which the health service intervention is for care rather than cure tend to have a lower profile.

Related to the above problem is the fact that health commissioners are under pressure to expend their resources in areas for which there is good evidence relating processes to satisfactory outcomes. This is a consequence of the cult of 'evidence-based medicine'. Again, conditions such as dementia in younger people are likely to be disadvantaged because the outcomes are less clear-cut, and there has been less effort expended on randomised controlled trials and other such rigorous studies. Furthermore, the nature of dementia makes such studies difficult. Alternative methodologies may be less acceptable to commissioners, particularly of health care.

Quality of available data

When performing population needs assessment, plentiful high-quality data is a considerable encouragement. In comparison with many conditions, the reliability of information from epidemiological studies of younger people with dementia is considered to be poorer. There is a mixed, and often poorly understood, aetiology to these conditions and a historical lack of adequate resourcing for high-quality studies of incidence and prevalence.

Adequate needs assessments also need good information about existing health and social services – changes are easier to make at the margin than at a 'zero base'. This process is much easier for acute hospital care where good information systems (as distinct from information technology systems) have existed for some time. The situation is different in areas dependent on community care. Deriving information on the strengths and dispositions of services in the community is fraught with difficulty. Despite much experimentation with various community information systems, there are still no adequate systems in the health service which can reliably inform commissioners as to what community care staff are doing, to whom, and at what cost. Commissioners are understandably reluctant to make marginal changes when they cannot see the margins clearly. It is recognised, however, that decisions may be driven by a variety of other factors, notably policy and cost, and that these may have significant impact, for example the closure of continuing care beds.

The lack of adequate information about care activity is similar for social care providers. Anecdotal evidence suggests that social care providers are still improving information systems in response to the community care reforms. However, there are still significant deficiencies, for example in terms of shared definitions. Among local authorities, many have different classifications of 'client group' with implications for the availability of information for comparisons and benchmarking, including the equity of provision between geographical areas.

Applicability of data from one population to another

There is likely to be a relatively small number of younger people with dementia in a planning authority's population, yet no easy access to reliable routine data on incidence and prevalence. To get round this problem, most authorities apply age- and sex-specific data derived from the small number of existing studies to their own populations. Implicit to this approach are the assumptions that, first, the only substantial determinant of the numbers of younger people with dementia in a population is the structure of that population and, second, that results derived from one population are generalisable to a completely different population. No account is taken of other factors which may have an impact on potential variations in incidence and prevalence, and scant regard is given to the important effect of random variation. This is particularly important for conditions where the number of individuals involved is likely to be small. Even when projected incidences are qualified by the use of 95 per cent confidence intervals, one commissioning authority in twenty is likely to have numbers outwith this band.

The population needs assessment approach is particularly suitable in areas where there is a clear association between the identification of the number of people affected and the services which they are likely to require. For instance, in assessing the needs of people with inguinal hernias, it is known that the majority of them will require relatively simple surgery which will cure their problems. Once the number of people are known, then the service requirements can be easily calculated. This is not true for dementia, nor indeed for the carers of people with dementia. Unfortunately, even if the number of younger people with dementia were known accurately, so diverse are their needs that it would be very difficult to derive a simple formula to calculate these needs, and the associated services required. Indeed, even if the specific needs are calculated, working out how to address them is complex.

Interaction between agencies

The role of population needs assessment is recognised as vital, particularly in community care, where many younger people with dementia live. Such assessment is a process involving agencies from health care, social care and the voluntary and private sectors. The information should inform service planning and delivery and ensure 'seamless care at home' (which by its nature must be planned and coordinated). Thus the process must be a joint one (SWSI 1996). While there have been a number of initiatives to encourage joint planning, such as the requirement for a joint community care plan produced collaboratively by health and local authorities, there are many fundamental differences between these organisations, for example in terms of culture, language, policy priorities and lines of accountability (SWSI 1996). Thus joint planning does suffer difficulties, such as the tendency for health authorities to concentrate their needs assessment work in areas for which the health service has main control and responsibility. Areas where there is a considerable input from social work services are understandably more complex and harder to tackle, in part because health services and social services have developed in different ways and have different perspectives on care.

Carers

In general, population needs assessments focus on the needs of the people with an identifiable disease, or who belong to a specific 'client group', rather than the carers who might provide the bulk of care and may be the sole reason for maintaining a person at home. However, supporting carers is vital for community care (e.g. DoH 1989). Thus there is a real need for information to plan and develop services for carers, yet the relatively limited information which does exist may not be suitable, for example the General Household Survey may allow estimates of the number of carers within population, and perhaps of their type (e.g. how many will be of what gender), but will not inform regarding the needs of this group.

The foregoing comments suggest that there are a variety of difficulties with top-down population needs assessment approaches to assessing the needs of younger people with dementia in the usual size of population considered by commissioning authorities.

Person-centred planning

Person-centred planning (e.g. Smale *et al.* 1993; SWSI 1996) approaches assessment in an interactive manner and aims to empower service users through a variety of features. These have been usefully summarised as an explicit value base, an attention to detail and process, and future orientation, a 'can-do' style, a commitment to user participation and/or representation (SWSI 1996). In essence, the thrust of the approach is to plan from the perspective of service users, with an attitude that challenges traditional assumptions, and with a commitment to seeking positive solutions.

It has been recognised that person-centred planning can contribute significantly to an understanding of both the needs of people and how they may be met (SWSI 1996). It should also be noted that all planning processes should rest on information; in the case of person-centred planning this information is often generated through the very process of planning itself, for example via involving service users. Such information will have a range of advantages (e.g. it is gathered directly from users) and disadvantages (e.g. it may not be representative and may be costly to gather). However, planning will always require robust, quantitative information, not least to estimate the numbers of people requiring and receiving care.

Discussion

Thus it may be seen that needs assessments for the population of younger people with dementia are difficult for a variety of reasons. There are significant difficulties in obtaining adequate information about such populations. Related to this, but a significant problem in its own right, are the prevailing attitudes of many providers (health, social work, voluntary sector and private sector) regarding younger people with dementia, and dementia in particular. Dementia is often regarded as something about which little can be done, and which will run its course no matter what intervention. However, while it is true that there is currently no cure for dementia nor universally effective treatments, interventions may have a wide range of profoundly positive effects, not least on the quality of life of the person with dementia and their carers and families. Greater awareness of the benefits of a range of interventions may affect the willingness of providers to address the needs of people with dementia, which in turn will drive a renewed incentive for better information.

In the meantime however, it is likely that planners for both health and social care will rely on historical provision as the basis for planning future services, yet such provision is often either inadequate or non-existent. Thus, when attempting to improve services, planners are faced with a lack of suitable information. The route out of such a difficult situation may involve two techniques: surveys and bottom-up approaches to information gathering. Such approaches may be applied to younger people with dementia and their carers, and be particularly useful for the latter.

Survey techniques have a number of advantages, for example they can in theory begin to identify the size of the population in question, though in practice this is likely to be difficult for younger people with dementia given the small number of such people and the potential effects of local variation. In addition, surveys may be expensive to conduct, requiring skilled staff for design, administration and analysis. However, a number of inroads into survey techniques have been made for people with dementia, including census techniques (e.g. Gordon and Spicker 1997). These can give a broad brush picture of the needs of a population which may be of utility to planners.

Bottom-up approaches seek to exploit the information already collected about the known, assessed population through aggregation, usually involving information technology. This has a number of advantages, including the detailed nature of such information and the potentially low cost of data collection. However, information is not available for the population which has not come into contact with services, and which may be experiencing significant unmet need. In addition, there may be issues surrounding the appropriate identification of the target population. Aggregated assessment information is of use only if the assessment tool is appropriate: as a minimum it must be quantitative, reliable and valid. In addition, it must be administered by staff skilled in the process of assessment.

The application of aggregated assessment information may become of greater importance given the likely encouragement which locality commissioning will receive. Evidence from one recent service development is encouraging (Cameron and O'Neill 1997; Cameron and O'Neill 1998). Nursing staff from one general practice use the Care Needs Assessment Pack for Dementia (McWalter *et al.* 1998) for individual needs assessments. The information is entered on computer to generate routine reports which are used as the basis for joint meetings with the local authority to plan care for those individuals. The information is available for aggregation, represents the needs of the known population, and may be used to contribute to the planning process for that area. While not devoid of problems (e.g. the difficulty of marrying planning for a practice population with diffuse geographical base and the defined geographical area served by the local authority) this represents one initiative to glean valuable information for planning from the process of delivering individual care on a joint basis.

Good needs assessment alone cannot result in good or even adequate services in any one area. There are a range of difficulties in the process of commissioning itself (NHS Health Advisory Service 1996) and further information may be required to complement needs assessment, for example a detailed knowledge of the services available from providers of health and social care, as well as those in the voluntary sector. However, a needs assessment based on both top-down and bottom-up approaches will provide information about both the incidence and prevalence of the condition, as well as more detailed evidence regarding the specific needs which the condition engenders, and at a local level.

Thus the assessment of need, of individuals and of populations, is a complex task. Each may require recourse to information from a range of sources, and each requires specific skills. A range of stakeholders, including service users and providers, is likely to have a legitimate interest, and may be included in the assessment and planning process in a variety of ways. Assessing the needs of younger people with dementia may be particularly difficult, for both individuals and populations, and for a variety of reasons. Yet progress in the practice of needs assessment could contribute to improved service delivery, and better services. Tackling some of these issues, for example the use of appropriate assessment tools, the wider adoption of the principles of good assessment, changing attitudes regarding dementia, and improving the information available to planners regarding this population, could result in improvements. In addition, further challenges lie ahead, notably incorporating that vital part of the skilled assessment – listening to the voice of the service user. Initiatives to address such a challenge will benefit from improved information about need.

Note: Further information about the Care Needs Assessment Pack for Dementia (CarenapD) (McWalter *et al.* 1998) is available from the Dementia Services Development Centre, University of Stirling.

CHAPTER 4

Opportunities and Threats
Multiagency Perspectives and Person-Centred Planning
Sylvia Cox

Introduction

The aim of this chapter is to review the opportunities and constraints which affect the ability of health and social care agencies to respond effectively to the needs of younger people with dementia and their support networks. Specifically, this chapter will:

- explore health and social support system responses to younger people with dementia

- identify some key issues in relation to interprofessional and interagency working and user and carer involvement

- indicate the scope for positive developments.

The chapter is based on development and consultancy work undertaken by myself with mainstream and specialist services, social work teams, primary care and multidisciplinary teams at both commissioning and service delivery levels in Scotland. It is also grounded in a development project at the Dementia Services Development Centre (DSDC) which explores the relationship between values, service objectives and outcomes from the perspective of the person with dementia. As a member of the working group which drew up the report on dementia as part of the Scottish Needs Assessment Programme (SNAP) established by the Scottish Forum for Public Health Medicine (SNAP 1997) I have been able to draw on a wider range of expert views. In much of this work, reminding people of the needs of younger people with dementia has often highlighted the ageist attitudes and patterns of service which so readily typify planning and service development for people with dementia generally.

Ordinary people with special needs

The particular grouping of signs and symptoms that are called 'dementia' depends not just on the level and severity of cognitive impairment, but also on the level and availability of social supports (American Psychiatric Association 1994). The pattern of social support for each person is different and is affected by a number of issues including:

- particular disease processes
- the unique individuality of the person concerned
- individual coping efforts
- availability of social support systems
- the response of wider society to their changing needs
- the quality, accessibility and appropriateness of available services.

Depending upon the individual combination of needs, strengths, social support and service responses, people with dementia, like others diagnosed with a chronic and life-threatening condition, have to find ways of living with this experience. Consequently, two complementary sets of needs emerge for the person themselves and those who act in the role of carer. First, to remain part of society. This will include continuing an ordinary life as long as possible, maintaining roles, responsibilities and interests. Others in their family and social network will have to accept their impairment and adjust to it whilst supporting them in their remaining strengths and abilities. Second, to have access to specialist help and services, as and when needed, from skilled and knowledgeable professionals and support staff who have a positive attitude to dementia and who are committed to developing and providing a range of health and social interventions and supports in a coordinated way.

Health and social care systems and practice may be well advised to reflect this dual focus. For a start they need to ensure that mainstream services – such as the primary care team, social work, housing, education, leisure, transport, health education, social security, legal services, the police, community pharmacists – are sensitised to the needs of all people with dementia; the emphasis here should be on social inclusion. Achievement of this aim involves multiagency and integrated approaches to health promotion, health and social education and community support. Moreover, health and social care systems need to spell out and publicise the linkage between mainstream services and specialist services, such as community mental health teams, dementia teams and specialist centres or memory clinics.

Whilst there is a shared perspective of people with dementia irrespective of their age, the implications of and responses to the two sets of needs described earlier may be distinctive. These include the increased likelihood of a fairly specific diagnosis, often at an earlier stage in its development, and the impact on roles and responsibilities associated with their particular stage in the life course, such as employment and family responsibilities. Additionally, younger people with dementia often fall between services for older people, people with mental health problems and other adult care groups such as those with physical and learning disabilities (Health Advisory Service (HAS) 1996). Therefore, the way that problems are experienced by younger people with dementia and their partners/families is crucially affected by their stage in the life course (Tindall and Manthorpe 1997) and the way that health and social care systems are set up to respond to their needs.

Significantly, younger people with dementia are beginning to be highlighted in government policy as an issue, though the implications for purchasers and providers are not very clearly spelt out (DoH 1997; Ministerial Task Force on Dementia Services in Victoria 1997). In Scotland, recent policy guidance includes specific references to younger people with dementia with regard to implementing services (Scottish Office 1997a). However, a recent survey by Barber (1997) of NHS Trusts in England confirmed that health services for younger people are provided within existing old age psychiatry services, although a third of the 304 trusts who responded (total 354) recognised the need to develop specialist services.

This underdevelopment is partly due to the fact that organisations do not usually respond well to diversity of need and relatively small needs groups. Health and social care agencies in the past have tended to approach the commissioning and purchasing of services in relatively large blocks and this has been influenced by the growth of the nursing home sector as an alternative to national health-funded longstay care.

This pattern is in spite of the underlying philosophy of the NHS and Community Care Act (DoH 1990) in the UK, which emphasised the importance of the individual within the overall process of care and assessment. However, on the other hand, the individualised approaches and care planning at the heart of community care offers an ideal way of responding to the range of issues encountered by younger people with dementia, regardless of their specific diagnosis or individual circumstances. Away from the UK other countries have also identified the importance of individualised care planning (Ministerial Task Force on Dementia Services in Victoria 1997), although a fundamental problem remains translating this principle into coordinated systems and practices.

Too often it is left to campaigning voluntary organisations and user groups to draw attention to particular areas of need such as Huntington's disease, HIV-related brain impairment (HRBI) and alcohol-related dementia. Thus the diversity and complexity of the types of dementia which may affect younger people has often led to fragmentation of services and marginalisation of needs. The fields of learning disability, Alzheimer's, HRBI, brain injury and other specialities have tended to develop their own areas of understanding, techniques, expertise and service developments. The UK Health Advisory Service thematic review on Huntington's disease, acquired brain injury and early onset dementia (HAS 1996, p.169) identifies these conditions as 'emblematic' of a whole range of brain disorders previously neglected by commissioners, purchasers and service providers. The report emphasises the importance of younger people with dementia as a special needs group because the people involved experience impairments which have an impact on all areas of life and often require significant and long-term commitments from health and social services as well as families. The current trend in health and social care policy to focus almost entirely on those with very high dependency needs or particularly challenging behaviour is also challenged: 'a service that is not provided early on can be a hidden source of expenditure later' (HAS 1996, p.2). Such an approach neglects the benefits of early intervention such as excluding treatable causes, enabling and supporting social networks, avoiding depression and anxiety, reduction of stress in carers (Ministerial Task Force on Dementia Services in Victoria 1997), also supporting the children of the younger person with dementia and young carers and giving genetic counselling where appropriate.

Much energy is also wasted by the separation of health and social care responsibilities. While it is crucial to understand and promote a social disability perspective on dementia, which focuses on normalisation and strengths, it is still necessary to recognise the need for skilled clinical, medical and nursing intervention. Younger people with dementia require skilled multidisciplinary assessment and they and their carers have continuing health care needs. Untreated physical and mental health problems may diminish the quality of life for the younger person with dementia and their family/social networks if they are not dealt with appropriately.

Accessing services

Most people, when they have a health or social care problem, turn first to family and friends for help and support; it is only if this is unavailable or does not provide acceptable reassurance, advice or assistance that they are likely to turn to outside agencies. The bulk of care in the community is provided by ordinary people, relatives, friends and neighbours, and much of the assistance which makes a real difference to people's lives comes from community-based resources. Obtaining the right kind of help depends upon the recognition and acceptance of problems in everyday living by the person themselves, or more often the person closest to them, such as family and friends or co-workers (Nolan, Grant and Keady 1996; Twigg and Atkin 1994). For younger people in the community, dementia is not often considered as a primary cause of difficulties. For people who have already been receiving services due to other conditions, such as learning difficulty, HRBI or alcohol problems, it can be just as difficult for professionals and care staff to acknowledge an underlying dementia.

Many services are constrained by a medical model of disability, rather than by one which encompasses a dynamic interaction of the biological, social and psychological factors. This view is often reinforced by health and social care systems which only see people at the point of diagnosis, crisis or failure of care systems; primarily breakdown of the situation at home, or a health crisis necessitating admission to hospital or nursing home. Concepts of empowerment and partnership between users and carers and service providers may not be considered in relation to younger people with dementia, not only because there are seen to be communication difficulties, but also because younger people with dementia are frequently not accounted for during consultative forums for user and carer initiatives, such as service planning and evaluation.

Excluding people from having an equal voice in society because they are disabled, whether physically or competency-based, has been a recurrent pattern in health care policy. Radical positive change has been most evident in the fields of people with learning difficulty, where those with very profound difficulties are seen as having the right to an ordinary life, particularly to their own home. However, people with mental health problems, people who develop a chronic or terminal illness and people with dementia have, until fairly recently, been excluded from these positive developments (Goldsmith 1996; Kitwood, 1997).

Deciding that help is required and then actually asking for it are not simple processes. For younger people with memory problems there are often fears about disclosing difficulties and the impact that this will have on others. In particular, asking for help from services primarily geared to older people can also be experienced as stigmatising. In an ideal world people need services that are discreet, supportive and tailored to their needs. The available options will thus depend on the accessibility of information about services, how easy it is for people to trust and share their problems and the quality of the staff and services involved.

A range of studies and reports have highlighted some positive aspects of existing resources and service systems, but on the whole have confirmed continuing carer and user dissatisfaction; mainly a case of 'too little too late' (Delaney and Rosenvinge 1995; Newens, Forster and Kay 1995; Quinn 1996; Sperlinger and Furst 1994). This was neatly summarised by a carer interviewed by Quinn: 'Well, as I say, the main thing is to have – for people to know about this illness and to get help straight away and not have all, you know, going from one place to another' (1996, p.27).

The distress of knowing there is something wrong can be compounded by social isolation, feelings of powerlessness and delays in getting a response or service. Such experiences may be cushioned by the involvement of a concerned general practitioner, a specialist mental health team, a sympathetic social worker or a community psychiatric nurse who make links with appropriate services and other professionals, provide ongoing practical and emotional support. All too often these appear to be isolated occurrences.

Pathways through dementia

The individual pathway through dementia is unique for each person. However, in order to plan effectively and to ensure integrated approaches to care planning and service development, the agencies involved may well need to identify common factors involved in both the clinical and care pathways. This approach is useful in service planning and commissioning as it enables services to identify the key service requirements and responses at each stage in the pathway (HAS 1996). The pathways approach is also a way of identifying the obstacles and supports for the individual's progression through services, a way of assessing quality and the achievement of user-led outcomes (Øvretveit 1993). The report by the Ministerial Task Force on Dementia Services in Victoria (1997) suggests that service developments can be usefully defined in response to:

- early difficulties
- emergence of significant difficulties in daily living
- reduced capacity for independence
- high dependence on care and incapacity.

Whilst there will be variations in the type and mix of problems, this modelling approach is important if existing services are to be redesigned or new ones developed. However, the kinds of pathways through systems will depend on the links between mainstream and specialist services, relations between community, specialist and hospital-based care, between health, social care, housing, the private, voluntary and statutory sectors.

For the younger person with dementia the main factors which affect the pathway are the:

- existing family and social support network
- access point into services
- stage in the development of the condition when the person is referred
- existence of another condition or disability e.g. learning disability, HIV
- urgency and complexity of problems.

For many people this experience seems like falling through the network of services rather than being supported by them and is captured in Figure 4.1.

The indicators of such a system are:

- emphasis on diagnosis and assessment as a one off occurrence
- emphasis on problems and clinical symptoms not quality of life and well being
- no integration or clear linkage between and within service systems such as health and social care, independent sector, housing and other community services
- poor or non-existent joint planning and commissioning of systems and services
- no contact person/key worker/case manager or continuity of professional support
- emphasis on weaknesses rather than strengths of family/person
- crisis-driven service responses

- pessimistic attitudes and little or no therapeutic input from professionals or support staff.

The causes of such a situation are many and various but may include poor strategic planning and joint commissioning work, poor information and communication systems, lack of continuity between mainstream and specialist service systems, uncertainty about who holds together review and service allocation, lack of awareness, knowledge and expertise in staff, lack of innovative and flexible services and sharing of good practice, fear of cost shunting

Falling through the net

Repeated contacts to GP…eventual referral to specialist (neurology/old age psychiatry/adult psychiatry) referred back to GP with diagnosis (not necessarily shared with person)… told will just have to manage to come back if there are problems…isolation, struggling on…deterioration…crisis in home situation…GP refers to social services…standard service – home care (non specialist), respite, day care (probably in older person's services)…daily living problems/possible challenging behaviour…home and day care services cannot cope…increasing levels of medication…referral to voluntary organisation…specialist day care/respite care/day hospital…person becomes more confused, withdrawn or challenging…family/carer becomes more stressed…carer asks for admission to hospital/nursing home…community care assessment carried out… provision of intensive domiciliary care…admitted to nursing home (older people)…possible later admission to acute hospital ward or continuing care… psychogeriatric ward or… different nursing home… for terminal care…

Figure 4.1 Falling through the net

between different parts of the system, particularly health and social care, acute and long-term services, poor monitoring and review of services and lack of vision and leadership.

Core values

However, there are perhaps more fundamental reasons why younger people with dementia do or do not receive appropriate services. These relate to the presence or absence of shared values across the different sectors which promote working in partnership with users, carers and social networks, empowering people to maintain responsibility and control, whilst mobilising additional resources which complement existing social supports.

Team work and effective collaborative working within organisations, between staff from different agencies, between professionals and users and carers can only be effective if there are explicit shared values and objectives, and if there is a consensus about what constitutes an effective outcome of service and the standards and quality to be achieved.

As discussed earlier, for the younger person with dementia the challenge is to hold on to the notion of ordinary life for as long as possible and to find ways of overcoming the loss of cognitive abilities. However, all too often there are difficult decisions to be made about the capacity of the person to sustain an acceptable quality of life in the community, and balancing individual rights to the, at times, conflicting needs of carers. A starting point to brokering a path between these conflicting interests could be the use of the biographical approach (Johnson 1986). In this model people with dementia are perceived as human beings who have led unique lives, and in their own individual ways are trying to cope with, and make sense of, a complex and profound change process. Personal accounts and research confirm that individuals need to 'hang on to' identity, meaning, awareness of self and others, but also to recognise loss and the need for interdependent support (Barnett 1997; McGowin 1993).

There are many approaches to the asserting of values and principles in relation to dementia (Kings Fund 1986) and at present the DSDC is exploring a framework of values which attempts to encapsulate the particular perspective of the person with dementia. This approach has been built up from existing research and quality systems and involves consultation with stakeholders, including users and carers. The approach attempts to promote the interdependency of the relationship between the person with dementia, their family and social network and wider society; drawing specific attention to meeting psychosocial as well as medical needs. In this way the DSDC framework emphasises the values of :

- maximising personal control
- enabling choice
- maintaining dignity
- preserving continuity
- promoting equity.

Consensus on values and principles is crucial because there may be conflict between stakeholders and interest groups which affect agreement on objectives, quality standards, priorities and resource allocation (Nocon and Qureshi 1996). Bringing together representatives of different stakeholders and involving users and carers in developing and commenting on the framework is one small way of involving people with dementia. Younger people are more evident in this process, partly because they are often more involved in understanding their diagnosis and aware of future implications, but also because they and their carers are less likely to be victims of ageism and exclusion and more able to challenge existing patterns of service provision.

Interprofessional and interagency working

A further factor influencing the pathway through health and social care systems is the way in which organisations, professionals and support staff work with each other. For example, the quality and effectiveness of service that users and their families receive is often due to the successful working between agencies and practitioners, especially in the field of younger onset dementia, because of the range of agencies and professionals involved. Multidisciplinary working involves professional practice issues as well as the organisational and structural relationships between agencies. It focuses attention on the way that professions work with each other to achieve appropriate outcomes for people who use services. These relationships are made more complex because of the involvement of support workers and direct care staff who provide much of the ongoing care and support to people in the community for people with mental health problems or dementia. The knowledge, skills, competence and not least attitudes of professionals and support workers are likely to have a significant impact on the effectiveness of multidisciplinary working.

In an area like dementia care where knowledge and ideas are changing so quickly, where there has often been a rather negative view of the potential for improvement or positive action, *specialist knowledge* is a key issue and an importance focus for interdisciplinary learning. This is especially true in relation to the needs of younger people with dementia where a range of specialisms may be involved. This specialist knowledge applied to particular individuals in specific situations may create opportunities for learning which can be shared at different levels with other professionals, support staff and users and carers.

Productive multidisciplinary working often involves a merging of roles and a preparedness to accept that another person is more appropriate and competent to carry out a particular task. This requires individuals to feel secure in their own professional identity and competence in order that they can accept advice from others. Networking, and informal approaches to multidisciplinary working can be very effective at a client level (Øvretveit 1993) and it is important that the emphasis on the need for better systems does not reduce this capacity by an overemphasis on top-down management. However, for this to happen there has to be agreement at joint planning and commissioning levels both within and across districts, otherwise services for younger people with dementia will not be implemented.

Interprofessional working often involves issues of power and status. Planners, managers, purchasers, providers, users and carers are likely to have different objectives and priorities. This set of complex dynamics can have a significant impact on the ability of agencies to achieve appropriate assessment, care planning, coordinated service delivery and outcomes with users of services. This is often most obvious on the boundaries between service systems where service managers are having to make difficult decisions about resource allocation and eligibility criteria, such as admission to nursing home care, and the level of costs for a community care package. Younger people with dementia are particularly vulnerable in such situations unless there are clear agreements between agencies about clinical and care pathways supported by positive and informed informal working relationships.

Partnership and positive pathways

The positive pathway set out in Figure 4.2 requires different agencies to work in partnership with each other and with users and carers to produce an integrated pathway. It is close to the spirit of community care (DoH 1990) but requires significant commitment and persistence on the part of those commissioning, managing and operating systems to become more responsive to the needs of the range of younger people with dementia and their families and carers. It may also involve cooperation across districts in the case of more specialist services.

The components of a more positive system have been broken down into the following five issues.

1. Sensitising the community and mainstream services to the needs of people with dementia of all ages

Generalist health and social care services such as housing, GP and community nursing care, home care services and carers services are usually the first point of contact apart from the person's own family and friends. Therefore they need information about the challenges posed by dementia as well as guidance on positive responses. Such responses include the importance of the person with dementia maintaining interests, skills, abilities, personal and social relationships and so on. Unless these frontline mainstream services are staffed by people who have some understanding of dementia, and that it can affect younger people, vital opportunities may be missed to help negotiate assistance.

Particular sensitivity is required in the early stages where there will be a range of possible contact points. The anonymity of helplines run by voluntary organisations may be preferred; a community mental health drop-in centre or a memory clinic may be more accessible if there are open referral systems; social services or community nurses may also be contacted depending on how the particular problem is identified. Some people may already be in receipt of services such as those for learning disability, HRBI or alcohol services and may already have a particular key worker or case manager (Alzheimer's Disease Society (ADS) 1996; HAS 1996), but these staff may not be aware of service developments in the dementia field. Development and consultancy work at the DSDC has revealed that it is possible in a locality for pockets of people with specific conditions, for example multiple sclerosis or Parkinson's disease and dementia, to be totally isolated from expertise and services in the dementia field.

2. Specialist multidisciplinary assessment

As we have seen in earlier chapters, diagnostic and assessment processes are entwined and complex. GPs need to call on specialist advice which may be available from local networks of specialists, depending on the problems involved, for example Huntington's disease and learning disability. These networks would need to be publicised amongst GPs, primary care teams and mental health teams if maximum benefits are to occur. Teams formed in this way may focus around a particular condition, and involve positive networking, collaborative work across health and social work, and professions allied to medicine, such as occupational therapy, physiotherapy, resulting in the sharing of expertise in particular conditions in particular localities. (ADS 1996; HAS 1996).

Memory clinics were mentioned in Chapter 1. These have traditionally been set up primarily for drug trials and have been poorly integrated into the network of services provided by health, social work and the private and voluntary sector. However, operating at their best level they are in a position to provide non-stigmatising and skilled diagnosis, and assessment, counselling and care planning. They also have the advantage in being an obvious focus for referral from both GPs and from users and carers themselves.

The HAS report (1996, p.87) suggests that very specialised centres should be available to serve populations of 2–3 million and distributed geographically. Multidisciplinary facilities are available such as those at the clinic for the counselling and diagnosis in dementia (CANDID) at The National Hospital for Neurology and Neurosurgery (Walton and Roques 1994), and the early onset dementia service described by Ferran et al. (1996). Such specialist centres, whether created by supplementing existing services or creating new ones, have a role in ongoing rehabilitation and support by providing teaching and training of key local staff, development of treatment approaches and techniques, research as well as assessment and interventions for individuals in specific cases. One of the key roles of specialist centres is to listen to the problems of local stakeholders and to ensure dissemination of clinical and care developments and research.

3. Multidisciplinary working

Community mental health teams are one model of providing a focus for multidisciplinary assessment, linkage with primary care and other specialist services and the ability to provide monitoring, review and intensive case management if required. However, they have not been without problems and have not necessarily included services for younger people with dementia. Often there was a concentration on less severe problems and an overemphasis on assessment and short-term intervention as opposed to longer term support and case management (Patmore and Weaver 1991). Wilcox et al. (1995) and Challis et al. (1997) evaluate the working of teams in relation to people with dementia, though not younger people. It is highly unlikely that people with dementia generally will be assessed and supported throughout the course of the disease by a community mental health team. Indeed younger people with dementia with diverse conditions may be more effectively supported through a client based network of professionals and support staff as long as there are clear arrangements for monitoring, liaison with primary care and the community mental health team. However, it would be helpful if community mental health teams developed a level of knowledge, expertise and skills in this area.

4. Individual care planning and support

The linkage between specialist assessment and community services is crucial. There is a danger that specialist multidisciplinary teams, whether at local or subregional level, merely 'prescribe' community care packages or a service solution such as day care, respite, residential care, the implementation of assessment and care.

Originating in England, the Care Programme Approach (CPA) has been seen as one way of ensuring:

- systematic assessment of health and social needs
- formulation of a care plan
- appointment of a key worker
- regular monitoring and review.

There appears to be a strong case for bringing together the CPA and the assessment and care management processes for younger people with dementia (HAS 1996). This would mean that each person had a named key worker/case manager in order to ensure continuity of care and access to assistance, particularly in cases of crisis or the need for 24-hour support. In many cases this would be a supportive/monitoring role, but could provide more intensive case management. Such arrangements would be essential where there were complex relationship and behavioural problems, for instance involving young carers or the likelihood of challenging or other high-risk behaviour. It may be useful for a care plan to be drawn up by a specialist team in conjunction with the person with dementia, carer/family network and key worker. An agreement could be made about follow up and review and incorporated within CPA with a close link to primary care services. It is important to keep open ease of referral back to the specialist service.

CPA may not be needed if skilled help from a full range of specialist and non-specialist services is available and there are good monitoring and review systems in place as well as access to intensive case management when needed. CPA in itself may not be sufficient, since effective programmes will often depend on the purchasing and implementation of appropriate services.

5. Intensive case management

Care management may be defined as the process by which care in the community is organised, delivered and financed in terms of the UK NHS and Community Care Act (DoH 1990). Care management may operate at different levels of intensity and with intensive case management being focused on specific types of cases. Opportunities to develop creative and workable care plans will depend on access to a range of resources which can be deployed flexibly.

The need to mesh together social work and mental health work along with the coordinating role of case managers across services and agencies was the crucial aspect of the service evaluated by Challis and colleagues in the Lewisham case management scheme (Challis et al. 1997). Although this study did not particularly address younger people with dementia it has pertinent comments about multidisciplinary working and systems of assessment and resource allocation. The identification of the significance of the case managers role at 'the interface between professional intervention and care work, which can be summarised as a combination of substituting for and relieving carers, providing specialist skills and sharing long-term responsibility' (Challis et al. 1997, p.148) seems particularly significant in relation to the type of interventions and service developments also appropriate for younger people with dementia. Such case managers have a crucial coordinating role across agencies and services.

It might be argued that younger people with dementia have such complex needs that following multidisciplinary assessment they should be offered an opportunity to have access to this kind of intensive case management service. Indeed, some of the specific services described in this publication have developed in this way (see Chapter 8 on alcohol-related dementia). Many of the staff involved in counselling services set up for younger people with dementia, whilst not acting directly as case managers, operate as facilitators and networkers with statutory and other voluntary and independent organisations. Such a pattern of service would involve the benefits of coordination as well as access to individually tailored services. Unfortunately, eligibility criteria for such intensive case management services often seem to relate not to the complexity of the need but to the immediacy of the risk of admission to hospital or residential/nursing home or a crisis situation with family carers; often producing interventions which are too late to be effective. However, many families will want to manage themselves, especially if they can get the appropriate professional, practical, financial and emotional support they need.

These five different components, when in place, can create a more positive pathway, as described in Figure 4.2.

The first requirement is a community sensitised to the needs of people with dementia, including younger people, so that there are positive attitudes to support. If the *first contact* is with a GP, primary care team or community service sensitised to the needs of younger people with memory problems and dementia, they are more likely to be referred to an appropriate *specialist team*

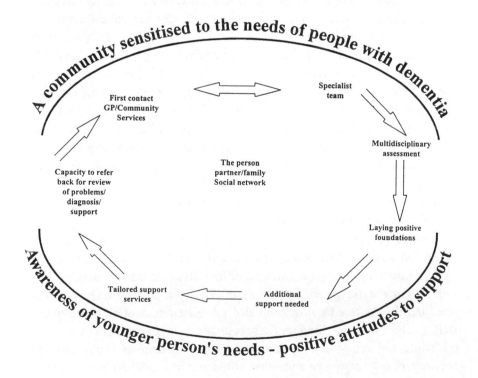

Figure 4.2 A circle of support

(this may be a subregional centre/specialist psychiatry unit/memory clinic or a learning disability, HRBI, alcohol-related specialist network). *Multidisciplinary assessment* should involve medical and nursing staff, social worker, psychologist and other relevant practitioners such as physiotherapist, occupational therapist, speech therapist, along with the person themselves and their partner/close relative/supporter.

Once a diagnosis has been shared, or indeed the need for ongoing assessment and review, steps can be taken by *laying positive foundations in the community*. Thus there is careful referral back to the GP or community mental health team. Ideally a named contact person or key worker is identified so that there is careful coordination of contact and the care programme. Negotiations can be made to plan for the immediate future, such as practical help in the home, therapeutic programmes, financial advice, counselling, work support. A contact phone number for an emergency or crisis should be given. Eventually, *additional support* may be needed. The requirement for intensive case management is dependent on the available support network but the agreed care programme should integrate diagnostic review, clinical treatment and social and individual support both for the person and the main carer.

Tailored support services should ideally be non-institution based, responsive, and based on individual knowledge. If there is a range of service options this will contribute to the maximisation of personal control, preserving continuity and enabling choice. Intensive support at home should not be left until the last resort and alternative forms of accommodation and support should be considered as early as possible if care at home seems problematic. Within the circle of support the *capacity to refer back for a review of problems/diagnosis* is essential, both to address particular problems or to revise the programme of care as needs develop, for instance in response to changes within the family or as the need for more intensive or palliative care arises.

Bringing it all together – person-centred systems and practice

How can this positive approach be translated into actual services on the ground which provide quality of life and care to people with dementia? Shared values and principles are essential if a person-centred approach is to be taken in providing programmes of care and support (Kitwood and Bredin 1992). The whole aim of such programmes is to enhance the quality of life for people with dementia and family (O'Brien, Pearpoint and Forrest 1993; Svanberg, Stirling and Fairbairn 1997). By promoting choice, decision making, meaningful activity and relationships, feelings of dignity, personal worth and something to share can be achieved. Some key principles are:

- that the person is treated in a holistic way, with a sense of his/her values, tastes, interests, abilities, strengths, spirituality
- a commitment to user participation and involvement
- that the person is accepted as part of a functioning social system with significant others who must retain a significant role
- that quality of life is determined in a range of ways which are meaningful to the person within his/her social system and community
- that the person is empowered to mould his/her own life as much as possible
- valuing the present but not denying the future – change and loss is accepted as an inevitable part of life
- a positive approach rather than pessimism
- an attention to detail and process in providing support and care
- biographical/lifecourse approaches and techniques.

Challis *et al.*, reviewing a range of studies addressing people with dementia (1997, p.142), identify two major issues which are also relevant to younger people with dementia:

1. Providing a standard range of services in terms of quality, volume and model, even if provided at an early stage, is not likely to enable people to remain at home or reduce carer stress to a marked degree.

2. Providing a more intensive service, providing substantially different services, targeted on those identified as needing additional support, especially if such services are different in quality and quantity, may have more impact.

Younger people with dementia often need additional support, and services that are different in terms of style and approach. There is a difficult tightrope to walk between ensuring that accurate, early differential diagnosis is made so that appropriate medical, therapeutic and social care for individuals is appropriately provided for younger people with dementia whilst not being drawn into stereotypical and stigmatising solutions.

Practitioners are particularly challenged by the lack of availability of innovative services for young people with dementia, such as family-based respite, work- or leisure-focused day activities, housing and support, since current arrangements make it difficult to purchase services that do not exist whilst commissioning new services requires a close relationship between those involved in identifying needs (users, carers and practitioners) and potential providers of services. This accentuates the point made earlier about the need for close working relationships between users and carers, care managers and service commissioners. Frontline staff are a significant factor in identifying and developing more responsive services. There may be advantages in close working between assessors and providers of services, especially where the needs of the user and/or carer are complex.

Such developments need also to take into account and respond more appropriately to language and cultural differences as experienced in black and ethnic minority communities (Brownlie 1991). Language, living environment, clothing, physical, social and spiritual care need to be consistent with the person's past identity and background, which may become even more significant as the person becomes more cognitively impaired. But it is not just about preserving the past, it is also about finding a way for new opportunities and experiences in a caring and supportive environment. Change may have to be managed, ideally in a gradual way that minimises stress and anxiety. Paid staff can be given guidance and support by relatives, friends and other community support systems to ensure consistency and continuity for people with dementia so that the services provided make sense in terms of their unique life history.

Conclusion

This chapter has highlighted the importance of both mainstream and specialist responses to the needs of younger people with dementia and those who care. This involves ensuring that health, social care and other community support systems provide integrated and accessible pathways to multidisciplinary assessment and service provision. Effective and high-quality systems rely not only on professional expertise, knowledge and skill, but on the dissemination and sharing of the practical application of such expertise with users and carers and non-specialist professionals and support staff.

Positive interagency and interprofessional working is required at planning, commissioning, system and practice levels if such developments are to become more generally available. User and carer involvement is also essential.

The acceptance of shared values across service systems is more likely to result in person-centred services and developments which address the individualised needs of younger people with dementia and those who care for them.

PART TWO

Specific Considerations

CHAPTER 5

HIV-Related Brain Impairment

Steve Jamieson

Introduction

This chapter focuses on HIV-related Brain Impairment (HRBI) and other changes to the brain sometimes associated with the human immunodeficiency virus (HIV). Brain impairment is a very distressing disorder for both patient and carer and it is one of the greatest fears of someone who is HIV positive. The intention of the overview is to inform not only nurses but also other professionals, support staff and others involved in the care of an individual with HRBI.

Attention is devoted to the medical definitions and historical context of HRBI before moving on to consider the incidence and prevalence of the condition. Management and care is then highlighted before addressing the future of services for people with HRBI.

Throughout the chapter the author draws upon his extensive experience in commissioning and developing HRBI units and implementing models of care to enhance a holistic approach.

HRBI: clinical characteristics

The diagnosis of HRBI often begins by the exclusion of any other possible causes of cerebral dysfunction. These include opportunistic infections, progressive multifocal leucoencephalopathy, brain tumours, other forms of dementia, depression and drug or alcohol misuse. Side effects of other medical treatments should also be considered such as peripheral neuropathy, delirium, or muscle damage. These are all common side effects of drugs used in HIV disease, such as AZT (zidovudine) and gancyclovir.

The most commonly presenting symptoms of HRBI are 'negative'; These include cognitive, social or motivational deterioration; memory loss; difficulty in walking; mental slowing; and depressive symptoms. These develop subtly over weeks and months, if not years. Less common presenting symptoms are tremor, behavioural changes, apathy, delirium and motor problems. Language function, attention and recognition are very rarely affected in the early stages. Close attention to all these features can often be used to distinguish those people who are using drugs or are depressed or anxious from those with early signs of HRBI.

However, there is a small but important subset of people who present with much more dramatic psychiatric symptoms, i.e. psychotic or manic states. Such individuals tend to come into contact with psychiatric or HIV services much more quickly because of sudden onset of, typically, what King (1993) calls an 'irritated mania' or acute confusion, recent onset psychosis or other signs of bizarre behaviour. Again, drug use and psychiatric history must be ruled out before a diagnosis of HRBI can be made. Often people with HRBI presenting with acute mania progress to a dementia type illness. El-Mallakh (1991) has suggested that there is a 'window of vulnerability' to psychosis or mania that occurs relatively early in the dementing process and that the progression to dementia is associated with the remission of the psychosis.

More typically, people with HRBI are not identified by either psychiatric or HIV services until much later in their disease progression because their symptoms are subtle and not recognised. As HRBI progresses, language and attention are affected and reading, writing and understanding language begin to deteriorate. In perhaps one- to two-thirds of people with HRBI, there is vacuolar myelopathy (a disorder of the spinal cord which causes difficulty in walking and incontinence). Severe apathy, psychomotor slowing and lack of insight are common in the later stages. Other common neurological complications are neuropathy and seizures. At a late stage in the illness the person is unable to walk and is doubly incontinent. Death usually follows soon after.

An early description of HRBI seen in AIDS was made by Navia and Jordan (1986) and Navia et al. (1986a,b). In these studies the authors presented detailed clinical and neuropathological data on a series of patients who had died of AIDS. Of the 121 patients in the sample, more than 40 per cent had some degree of cognitive impairment caused by disease of the central nervous system (CNS) secondary to their HIV infection. In addition, more than a third of this group showed some cognitive or behavioural changes for which, at that time, there was no explanation. From the medical records of this group, Navia et al. were able to describe a triad of clinical features which they later labelled the AIDS dementia complex (ADC). The triad consisted of *cognitive impairment* (including forgetfulness, loss of concentration, confusion and slowness of thought), *motor dysfunction* (including loss of balance, leg weakness, deterioration in handwriting) and *behavioural changes* (including apathy, social withdrawal, organic psychosis and regressed behaviour). Most of the patients with HRBI had a pre-existing diagnosis of AIDS ($n = 29$), but in 17 cases, HRBI had developed in people who were otherwise well. Although there have been many reports of dementia being the first manifestation of AIDS (Navia and Price 1987) this is relatively uncommon (McArthur *et al.* 1989). The Centres for Disease Control (CDC) criteria for a diagnosis of AIDS now include dementia as an AIDS-defining syndrome (CDC group IV). This means that, by definition, it is no longer possible for a person with a symptomatic disease to have dementia.

Terminology and concepts

The concept of the AIDS dementia complex has been developed by Price and Brew (1988) to include a clinical rating scale that has been widely used in research studies. The ADC scale allows individuals to be rated on one of six levels from normal (Stage 0) through equivocal (Stage 0.5) to end stage dementia (Stage 4). Ratings are made by comparing a patient's clinical presentation with descriptive exemplars.

Navia and Jordan's (1986) clinical description of the cognitive and behavioural changes seen in advanced HIV disease has been widely accepted. The use of the term 'ADC', is more controversial. One of the major criticisms is that the term 'complex' and behavioural changes necessarily go together. From Navia and Jordan's report, it is clear that some individuals displayed evidence of either motor or cognitive impairment without the other features of the ADC triad. The use of the term 'dementia' has also been challenged.

Although ADC is one of the more widely used diagnostic categories to describe the cognitive and behavioural changes sometimes seen in AIDS, at least 12 other labels are used to describe a variety of similar clinical presentations. In an attempt to rationalise the terminological confusion, the World Health Organization (WHO; 1990) recommended the adoption of a new diagnosis, 'HIV-1 associated dementia', based on operationally defined criteria adapted from the ICD-10 diagnosis of dementia. To achieve a diagnosis of HIV-1 associated dementia the ICD-10 criteria for dementia must be met with the following modifications: (1) the decline in memory may not be severe enough to impair activities of daily living; (2) motor dysfunction may be present; (3) aphasia, agnosia and apraxia are uncommon; and (4) the symptoms should have lasted for at least one month. Further to this, the patient must be HIV seropositive and other possible aetiologies should have been excluded.

The WHO diagnostic system has several disadvantages.

1. It realigns the use of the term 'dementia' with its use in other diseases such as Alzheimer's.

2. It plays down the importance of the non-cognitive and motor aspects of the disorder which, although common, are not always seen.

3. It emphasises the importance of excluding other causes of cognitive impairment that may occur in AIDS. This point is of great clinical importance as some CNS diseases are treatable (e.g. toxoplasmosis) whereas a diagnosis of dementia is often taken to suggest that nothing can be done.

Prevalence of HRBI

HIV has been found in the brain just two days after HIV infection (Bowen, Lane and Franci 1986) and over 90 per cent of people dying from AIDS have some evidence of brain damage on autopsy.

This is generally non-specific or from opportunistic infections. Even though the virus is present in both the brain and spinal fluid from soon after infection to death, the question remains how many people will then develop symptoms of HRBI.

An early study by Grant and Atkinson (1987) suggested that up to 44 per cent of HIV positive but asymptomatic patients had significant neurological dysfunction. This small study had a significant impact and was, in part, responsible for the screening of so-called sensitive personnel in certain sections of the United States military. In the United Kingdom the incidence rate is 7 pre cent. Later, more reliable studies, suggested that less than 1 per cent of asymptomatic seropositives develop dementia, with that figure rising to up to 20 per cent of people with overt AIDS. In other words, people with high CD4 counts and low viral loads rarely get severe cognitive problems. HRBI has increasingly become a part of the later HIV disease picture.

There is some research to suggest that the frequency of HRBI has been lowered considerably since the introduction of AZT. However, McArthur and Hover (1993) point out that the overall incidence of HRBI in the multicentre AIDS cohort study in the US changed over the last six years. This has to be put into the context of people living longer with better treatments

for other illnesses; perhaps it is evidence that anti-retroviral agents have sta-
bilised the incidence of the condition.

In children with HIV, the most commonly reported finding is neurological deterioration; around 50 per cent of children with AIDS have progressive
encephalopathy. The picture is different in children in that they are likely to
fail to meet their developmental 'milestones' or have normal neurological
development. In fact, the strongest evidence for the efficacy of AZT in the
brain comes from studies in children (Bowen, Lane and Franci 1986).

Neuropsychiatric implications of HIV for nursing care

This section mainly addresses the nursing needs of people with HRBI,
although the philosophy of care remains applicable to other groups. While
impairment of cognitive ability in people with HIV and AIDS has been
widely reported, the number of people either seriously or mildly affected is
not known. Regardless of numbers, nurses are increasingly having to assist
people who have cognitive dysfunction associated with HIV/AIDS.

Impaired cognitive functioning may involve problems with:

- reasoning
- memory
- judgement
- orientation
- perception
- attention
- concentration.

These are the processes which allow an individual to make sense of experience and to interact productively with the environment.

Impaired cognitive functioning leaves the affected person in a state of
confusion, unable to understand their experience, unable to relate current to
past events, to exercise judgement, to make decisions or to orientate
him/herself to time and place. The dysfunction may result in, or contribute
to, a number of needs/problems requiring assistance from nursing staff.
These include:

- *depression*: anxiety, personality changes; confusion; apathy; loss of motivation
- *irritability*: perceptual disturbance, restlessness; mood swings; disturbed sleep pattern; social withdrawal

- *loneliness*: social isolation; impaired functioning in work; interference with daily activities; neglect of personal hygiene; lowered self-esteem.

An adequate knowledge base

A clear understanding of the many neuropsychiatric or neuropsychological manifestations of HRBI will enable nurses and other care providers to maximise their techniques and skills in caring for people with the condition. It assists them in making appropriate referrals at the right time. Even if the dementia itself cannot be halted, many associated conditions respond well to appropriate treatment.

Familiarity with the relative merits of assessment tools available sharpens up the assessment of the needs and problems of patients. A vital aspect of this is that proper assessment provides a baseline from which the success of future nursing interventions can be measured.

Sensitive communication

The ability to communicate sensitively is the core of providing nursing care to a patient with cognitive impairment. Communication may be difficult because of confusion, forgetfulness, wandering attention, withdrawal and unresponsiveness, emotional lability, slowness of thought processes and impaired judgement in understanding what is socially acceptable.

Useful approaches/interventions

The following points give some indication of useful approaches:

- plan and allow enough time for interaction and the consequences
- assume there is capability for insight – check for understanding; do not be patronising or use ritualistic expressions
- record specific interventions that seem to work for particular people and particular situations; build upon knowledge and skills together
- try to have someone observe your conversation, both verbal and non-verbal
- encourage feedback, make suggestions, swap ideas; use these ideas/observations for educational purposes; make use of role play
- become familiar with reality orientation techniques and validation therapy; try them out; be purposeful in your interaction

- if you say you are going to do something, DO IT; if you forget re- turn to the person and apologise – do not assume that because you have forgotten, then the other person has too.

Self-awareness and the right attitudes

The nurse's most important attribute is his/her attitude. Regardless of the impairment, the person is entitled to be treated with respect and dignity. Looking after people who are confused, prone to mood swings, irritable and angry can be demanding and frustrating. Research has shown that nurses often react by avoiding contact with such people. To be effective, nurses need to be aware of the effects of such behaviour on themselves. They need to acknowledge that they can be angry, frustrated and hurt. Such feelings must be seen as natural and not a weakness. They must not be punished but expressed and dealt with appropriately either in staff support groups or supervision. Support and supervision is not a luxury. It is a vital part of the work of the nursing team.

Care needs

The impact of being infected with HIV often results in a variety of mental health problems which can be exacerbated by the onset of HRBI. There is also a range of very specific care needs.

As a result of HIV affecting the central nervous system clients may be:

- impaired in their ability to self-care
- a danger to themselves and/or others
- at risk of their condition worsening through lack of appropriate in- terventions.

There are also a range of physical needs requiring both occupational and physiotherapies to improve mobility and the ability to perform very simple tasks.

Clients therefore require a range of services to:

- enable them to remain as independent as possible yet safe from rea- sonable harm
- feel familiar and relaxed in their surroundings
- feel supported in times of distress
- feel supported in their possibly deteriorating condition.

As with all people with an AIDS diagnosis there is an ever present risk for people with HRBI of contracting another AIDS related illness requiring acute in- patient care. Lay and professional carers should be vigilant and have expertise in identifying any features that might indicate a change in the medical needs of the client. Given the rapid onset of HRBI and its relatively poor prognosis the need for high care is only likely to last for a short time.

Carers' needs

It is often the case that the needs of a distressed carer come to the fore in cases of HRBI. The needs of carers include:

- the need for support and advice, including details of prognosis and likely course of the illness
- respite from providing care to the partner, friend, family member
- advocacy to negotiate in care planning, legal matters and employment issues
- practical help and support to deal with various activities of daily life.

In summary, the development of services for this client group should include services for informal carers. Many people have very committed carers who require adequate support. In developing these responses consideration should be given to the need for confidentiality and the potential for this to be breached as a result of a client's loss of awareness. Multiple bereavements are a factor in HIV given the specific communities affected and this in turn creates further mental health problems. There is also an issue of double stigma affecting people with HRBI given the prejudice associated with mental health problems.

The use of generic, specialist and mainstream services

Services in this area can be described as a continuum of degrees of specialism:

- specialist HIV provision where the expertise is focused solely on people with HRBI
- mental health teams within HIV provision where the expertise includes experience in a wide range of mental health problems associated with HIV
- community HIV teams who are skilled in providing a range of HIV care for clients in their own home
- generic HIV centres which provide a range of treatments or services to clients with HIV, including community-based voluntary sector projects and acute HIV care centres

- mainstream mental health providers, both community-based and hospital-based, local and health authority, i.e. psychiatrists, psychologists, community psychiatric nurses and psychiatric social workers; the role of home care staff and the direct caregivers should also be included

- specialists working in the field of dementia and mental health offering advice, advocacy, supported housing and nursing home care.

In exploring the possibility of accessing mainstream and/or non-HIV services for this client group there are a range of possible hurdles. Professionals need to be able to assess any changes in care needs that may be caused by the onset of an AIDS-related complication in order to be able to refer it on appropriately. Following the move towards community care and the fairly recent closure of many of the large mental health hospitals, the mainstream services are stretched to capacity and not adequately meeting demand.

Models of care

A number of approaches are applicable to this client group that stand alone as distinct models of care. In practice they represent the total range of available services and are linked to provide packages of care.

Home support

This provides care for a person in their own home and comprises of a range of services usually coordinated via social services, the community trusts and in some cases, the acute care centre. The care is designed to enable a client to remain at home. The care might be managed by the person's GP and will comprise of up to 24-hour constant nursing/auxiliary care.

Floating support

This model offers clients a similar style of service to intensive housing management schemes although the person is living in ordinary housing; support is usually less intensive. The advantages are a higher degree of flexibility, since it can be offered to people in privately rented, owner-occupied and housing association property and it tends to be more cost effective.

Day care/day activities

Clients are referred to day care from any of the above facilities to provide a structured programme of care designed to meet their needs, in relation to their cognitive impairment, their physical incapacity and their behaviour changes.

Short-term residential care

This is available in a range of facilities which are either nursing home or hospice based. It is designed to provide care for a person at times of increased need but where their primary residence remains their own home. This can be offered on a rolling respite scheme where short stays are planned in advance on a preventative basis.

Palliative/hospice-based care

This care provides symptom control, terminal care and a range of other therapies which may include complementary, nutritional and occupational therapies. There is also a community-based hospice service to provide ongoing care at home.

Long-term residential care

Such care includes residential, nursing and small group homes where most care and support is provided on the same site. Patrick House, a residential unit for people with HRBI, was opened in 1991 in West London, however it was closed in 1997 due to money being spent on combination therapies instead. Other similar services are being developed but the balance between high standards of care and costs remains an issue for those people who do require alternative nursing care in a residential setting.

Acute in-patient care

In relation to clients with HRBI, acute care is needed for assessment, initial treatment, and to treat the onset of any other AIDS-related illnesses.

The relative advantages of each of these models of care vary. They have all been found to be of some benefit as part of a total package. Each can be designed to address the specific needs of this client group, in relation to emotional, medical, social and spiritual needs. Obviously the balance will vary, dependent upon a service being more socially or medically based or where the spiritual needs are paramount.

In the residential care of patients who have more severe brain impairment where their behaviour is noticeably affected with disinhibition or mania, there are two differing approaches:

- an integrated approach where patients are cared for on wards dealing with a variety of disorders

- an approach where clients are cared for in a separate setting to enable more specialised care and to avoid exposing other people to their more disturbing behaviour.

- A range of residential and day care provision
- Supported housing
- Home care packages
- Shared care including both primary and acute care
- Multidisciplinary teams
- Acute provision – specifically for early diagnosis, appropriate preventative and ongoing treatment, acute care, assessment, palliation and stabilisation
- Legal and social support
- Good links with generic services
- Links with specialist HRBI and/or HIV mental health services
- Respite and ongoing support for carers
- Rolling respite for users as a preventative measure

These services should all be adequately and appropriately resourced, financially, with training and support. Coordination and collaboration are vital, as is some form of directory/database to be regularly updated. Access to specialist knowledge and expertise is also essential.

Figure 5.1 Components of good service provision for this client group

The factors to be considered when assessing efficacy are as follows:

- the importance of moving away from a purely medical model of care to ensure that the clients are cared for in a holistic way; this needs to take account of the poor prognosis, the degree of possible deterioration, the impact of the illness on the clients underlying emotions and the lives of those around them

- the need for ongoing assessment of any changing medical needs to provide for appropriate treatment

- the need to balance a client's independence with potential risk to the safety of themselves and those around them
- the value of matching the care provided to the client's specific needs regarding adequate structure, familiarity, stimulation and support
- the need to take account of any complicating factors when planning care and to be as flexible as possible.

The relative cost effectiveness of each model of care is hard to assess unless the different parts of the care package are included.

Good practice in HIV dementia care

Improving the quality of care for people with dementia and their carers can be a great challenge. There should never be any one standard method of providing services to people with dementia. The basic rights and needs of people with dementia include human value, variation in human need, individuality and the non-exploitation of carers. Practical services are needed to turn these principles into reality for people with HIV related dementia and their carers.

Staff training and support

Much is said in the literature about the issue of so-called 'burnout' of staff in the HIV and AIDS field. It is in the employers' and staff's interests to ensure that this is addressed and measures are put in place to deal with the stress of dealing daily with the often tragic circumstances of people with AIDS.

The second issue that arises is that of homophobia. Since the appearance of AIDS there has been increasing concern about prejudice against homosexual people and reports of hostility on the part of health professionals towards homosexuals persist. Since at least 1988, gay and lesbian groups, including doctors, have been highlighting the problems in the health services for homosexual people and the psychological consequences of this type of discrimination. Indeed, because of the problems or perceived problems that many homosexuals face with what they regard as a homophobic medical establishment, some evidence points to their preference for doctors and nurses who are themselves gay.

Client empowerment/autonomy

Empowerment of clients should be considered important as long as their own safety and that of others is not jeopardised. Autonomy or personal control is also considered important, although rights have always to be balanced with responsibilities.

Reliability, consistency and quality of service

A reliable and consistent service helps to build trust with clients and carers. From clinical developments undertaken by the author, good practice relates to staff working in small teams with the ability to multitask and 'cover' for each other. It is also vital that people with positive attitudes are recruited and that they are encouraged to stay by offering reliable, consistent, quality salaries, training, supervision and support.

Mixing clients

Residential services encourage mixing of clients with different levels of cognitive impairment and aetiologies but also require facilities where people exhibiting displays of challenging behaviour could be temporarily accommodated. People with HIV but no dementia may need a great deal of support in this type of environment. There are also possibilities for cross-fertilisation of staff skills and ideas in residential care. In the author's experience, social service managers often believe that the behaviour and quality of life of people in residential homes improves by mixing with non-residents (for example with day care clients) and that non-residents lose their fear of residential care. However, evidence remains inconclusive as to the relative merits of the practice and may depend on how the service is managed and supported.

Assessment

An assessment should always be made after referral, although some services question the need to include the partner, relative or carer, which may cause difficulties.

Admission / discharge policies

If a client is to be admitted to a residential home it is considered good practice to arrange a pre-admission visit to a residential centre. This helps the individual to feel safer and allows them to express their opinion on the centre. This same approach may be relevant to day and respite centres. There should be no gaps between discharge and the start of the next service provision. This provides consistency for the client and reduced uncertainty for the carer.

Care teams

Care teams should be multidisciplinary and have clear boundaries and good communication with both mainstream and specialist services.

Care plans

Care plans should be individualised, reviewed frequently and involve good communication between all involved. Contingency plans reduce uncertainty and anxiety.

Techniques used to support clients should be variable, although those often used are mainly traditional: reality orientation, validation, life review and music therapy. Perhaps other, more creative, models could be considered.

People with HRBI can retain insight quite far into the dementing illness and it is therefore not surprising that some people often show challenging behaviour in an attempt to communicate their needs. Good neuro-psychosocial assessments (including psychometric testing) are essential and lead to better understanding of this behaviour.

Involvement of the carer, partner and family is very important, taking into account issues of confidentiality and relationships.

Design of accommodation

Accommodation for a person with HRBI should be adapted as little as possible from a traditional domestic home and should reflect the resident's individual needs. However, there are increasing examples of incorporating some dementia design principles into accommodation for people with HRBI.

Ideally, as in other models of dementia care, numbers should not exceed groups of four to six residents (unlike traditional nursing and residential models). More than this number may mean that staff are deployed to support the needs of higher dependency clients whilst those with lesser needs receive inadequate attention.

Support for care workers

Stress amongst volunteers and staff working with people who have AIDS is rife. This is often a result of overinvolvement and attachment with insufficient support. Without support, staff can feel hopeless, pessimistic, ambiguous about their role and futile when a client dies. 'People work' requires that staff be supported at two levels: first, the basic worth of work must be acknowledged by both peers and managers, and second, there must be explicit recognition of the emotional impact of caring.

Supervision (both managerial and clinical), performed by trained supervisors can support people to work with the 'everyday' frustrations, anger and sadness that workers describe. The losses involved with dementia and the multiple deaths that a worker may exercise in the HIV field must be supported as all of the other losses that a worker has experienced in their life will be touched upon following a death. Only when care workers and carers are really listened to and given help to increase awareness of their own thoughts and feelings, can they give good care.

Conclusion

With the advent of effective combination treatment, individual life expectancy in HRBI has increased. Evidence of direct HIV brain infection, combined with the knowledge that the brain becomes infected early in the course of systemic HIV disease, has stimulated efforts to find anti-retroviral drugs which can penetrate the blood-brain and blood cerebral fluid (CSF) barrier. AZT has this property. It is no longer the only anti-retroviral therapy available but the efficacy of new agents in the treatment of HRBI needs to be established, for example dideoxyinosine (DDI) and dideoxycytosine (DDC). There are some preliminary reports concerning the treatment of dementia using DDI but DDC is unlikely to be effective as it does not cross the blood-brain and CSF barrier.

Incidence of HRBI is increasing and this may be due to combination drug therapies extending life expectancy. At present hospices are having to diversify their services to cope and are frequently employing psychiatric nurses to assist. At the end of the last decade the Royal College of Psychiatrists (1989) commissioned a report on HIV/AIDS and psychiatric practice, which made four recommendations. These were:

1. Each mental health unit should address the psychiatric implications of HIV infection by ensuring that all staff are aware of the range of psychiatric problems likely to occur, and the possible effect of patient care and organisation of services.

2. All staff should be aware of the practical aspects of infection control as well as the ethical and legal issues that arise in the context of HIV infection. This can best be achieved by developing educational programmes at local levels.

3. Specific policies related to the needs of each mental health unit may need to be developed in collaboration with the policies established in the health district and at national level.

4. Psychiatrists should ensure that local health planning takes into consideration the likely psychiatric implications of HIV/AIDS infection.

The issues for the future of HRBI is that it is on the increase and with the introduction of combination therapy we are unable, at present, to confidently predict the epidemiology of the condition.

At a time of competing demands within the health and social care services, the need for a coherent policy is urgently required. It is hoped that this chapter has taken a few small steps in mapping out a suitable direction.

CHAPTER 6

Huntington's Disease

Roseanne Cetnarskyj and Mary Porteous

Introduction

This chapter is intended to help the reader understand that families affected by Huntington's disease (HD) have all of the problems associated with the care and understanding of other young people with dementia. In order to explain the complex needs of HD families, it is necessary to give a brief explanation of what HD is and how it is inherited.

What is Huntington's disease

HD is a genetic disease which can affect both men and women. HD interferes with the individual's ability to function physically, mentally (cognitively) and emotionally due to a deterioration of specific areas within the central nervous system. Symptoms usually first appear when an individual is between 30–45 years old but about 5 per cent of people show symptoms under 20 (commonly known as Juvenile HD) and another 5 per cent do not show symptoms until they are over 60 (Scottish Huntington's Association 1996).

If an individual (male or female) has the HD gene they will at some point in their life develop HD and any child of that individual will have a 50 per cent chance of inheriting the HD gene. To explain this further, we all have two copies of each gene and if an individual has the faulty gene they can pass on either their faulty copy or their good copy. If an individual does not inherit the faulty gene they will *not* develop HD nor will they pass it on to their children. Although in some families HD may appear to skip a generation, this is because the apparently unaffected individual has died before developing symptoms.

The first sign of HD is very variable: some people present with restless legs, some with a depressive illness or psychosis, and others with cognitive impairment. Despite each person's illness developing and progressing differently, they will have many similar symptoms. A particularly good description of the onset of HD is given in the handbook produced by the Huntington's Society of Canada:

> Early symptoms may appear as slight physical, cognitive or emotional changes. Physical symptoms may initially consist of 'nervous' activity, fidgeting, a twitch in the arms or legs, or excessive restlessness. The individual may notice a certain clumsiness, alteration in their hand writing, or difficulty with normal daily physical skills such as driving. These initial motor symptoms will gradually develop into more marked involuntary movements such as jerking and twitching of the head, neck, arms and legs, which may interfere with walking, speaking and swallowing. There are, however, exceptions to this. Sometimes people with HD have a minimum of difficulty with chorea (involuntary movements). Where chorea is present, the movements usually increase during voluntary effort, stress or excitement, and tend to decrease during rest. In addition to the early physical symptoms of HD, there are often very subtle cognitive signs as well. These may involve little more than a reduced ability to organize routine matters or to cope effectively with new situations. There may be the loss of short-term memory which may occur several times each day. Work activities may become more time-consuming. Decision making and attention to detail may be impaired. Early emotional signs may be equally subtle. These may be an accentuation of certain aspects of the individual's normal make-up such as more periods of depression, apathy, irritability, impulsiveness or there may be a change in their personality. (Huntington's Society of Canada 1996, reproduced with kind permission)

The disease commonly progresses slowly over a period of 15–25 years. Not everyone will exhibit all the physical, mental and emotional features of HD. This variation is one of the major causes of inadequate service provision. There is a danger of professionals with limited experience of HD making inappropriate generalisations about the needs of other HD patients based on the experience of one or two cases.

HD is caused by an enlargement or expansion in the Huntington gene located at the tip of the fourth largest chromosome. The expansion alters the gene function leading to damage or death of the nerve cells in certain areas of the brain.

The HD gene was identified by scientists working as part of an international collaboration in March 1993. This breakthrough has led to many research projects throughout the world aimed at identifying the normal function of the gene and the change associated with the expansion so that progress can be made towards a treatment to ameliorate or cure HD.

The worldwide prevalence of HD is 5–10 per 100,000. This figure is supported by the results from prevalence studies in South Wales in 1971 (7.61 per 100,000; Harper 1996) and 1981 (8.85 per 100,000; Quarrell *et al.* 1988), East Anglia in 1971 (9.24 per 100,000; Caro 1977), and in Grampian in 1984 (9.95 per 100,000; Simpson and Johnston 1989). A wide selection of prevalence studies can be found in Harper (1996, p. 213).

Testing available for HD families

Since the discovery of the gene in 1993, clinical genetic services departments throughout the UK and internationally have been able to offer a direct gene test to individuals who are at risk of HD. Three tests are available for HD families: confirmation of diagnosis, presymptomatic gene testing and prenatal diagnosis.

Diagnosis

If a doctor suspects an individual has HD he/she can discuss this with the patient and offer the test to confirm or refute the diagnosis. This should always be done in conjunction with the family and the implications for the family discussed should the diagnosis of HD be made.

Presymptomatic gene testing

In the UK, the UK HD Prediction Group aim to monitor all centres offering the HD test and encourage the use of a minimum protocol. Each centre's protocol will vary slightly but should fall within the consensus guidelines. The group recommends testing should only be offered to individuals of 18 years and over as HD is an adulthood onset disease with no effective treatment available. At present about 10 per cent of those at risk choose to be tested. This will no doubt increase if a treatment or a cure for HD is developed. The protocol for testing described in Table 6.1 is used in the South East of Scotland Clinical Genetic Centre. Individuals undergoing testing are encouraged to bring someone to each visit for support.

Table 6.1 Protocol for testing for HD

Visit	With whom	Time lapse	Content
First	Consultant geneticist		Discuss reasons for testing and confirmation of family history
Second	Clinical nurse specialist	2–4 weeks	Completion of questionnaire
Third	Consultant psychiatrist	2–6 weeks	Discussion of coping strategies
Fourth	Consultant geneticist	2–4 weeks	Consent and taking of blood
Fifth	Consultant geneticist	2 weeks normally – exact date given at fourth visit	Result given verbally and in writing
Post result	Consultant geneticist	usually 1 month	as discussed/ dependent on result

The UK HD Prediction Group state that an adult at 25 per cent risk can be tested even if their 50 per cent risk parent has chosen not to be tested; i.e. the person at 25 per cent risk's right to know their status overrides their parent's right not to know their status.

Exclusion of gene by foetal testing

Pre-exclusion testing on a foetus is also available for 50 per cent risk individuals, either those who do not want to know if they have the gene but only want to have a baby who is not carrying the gene, or to gene carriers who wish to have a baby which does not carry the gene. These tests should be discussed with the geneticist prior to becoming pregnant or as soon as possible after confirmation of the pregnancy, as they involve complex decisions and accurate timing.

Information on all tests can be obtained from any local genetic department and it is advisable to be in contact before considering any of the testing procedures to avoid decisions being made on wrong information.

HD and dementia

Dementia is a common and debilitating component of HD, although one major and important difference between the dementia in HD and other early onset dementias is that a person with HD does NOT lose recognition of their close family and friends.

When HD is diagnosed the diagnosis has a direct effect on everyone in the family. Whilst this is true of the impact of dementia on any family, HD as a genetic disease causes particular strains. The person with HD has to live with the knowledge that their children are at 50 per cent risk. Many partners of a person with HD live with the knowledge that they may have to care for their adult child with HD after many years of caring for a partner. It has also been known for a spouse to be caring for their partner and their adult child at the same time. 'It is not uncommon for a person to nurse their parent, then an older brother or sister and then finally succumb to the disease themselves, while worrying all the time that they have transmitted it to their children.' (Health Advisory Service (HAS) 1996, p.38). At diagnosis the brothers and sisters of the person with HD are confronted with a 50 per cent risk of having the gene themselves. A diagnosis of HD can cause family rifts as each family member chooses to confront or deny the disease. Many families have been known not to allow the children – i.e. cousins – to have contact with each other for fear that they could discover their risk of HD.

Challenges early in the disease process

This can be one of the most distressing times for HD families. Many of the physical signs of HD are not present, but cognition has deteriorated and emotional symptoms may be obvious to the family but not to others. Outsiders may think the person has become strange or has a drink problem as speech may become slurred and memory poor. During this period of the illness many families report lack of support, understanding and information from professional staff. It is also during this time the family of the person with HD may have to cope with their relative denying there is any problem, despite there being problems at work, in their social life, or their having several small car accidents. (When a person is diagnosed with HD they must inform the car insurance company or their policy will become null and void.) Due to denial or lack of understanding of the implications of the illness the person with HD may have to endure workplace disciplinary procedures and lose employment, but with sensitive negotiations this can be prevented.

With the new Disability Employment Act the employer can be advised and supported and in many cases employment can continue, adding to the well being of the employee with HD. Time needs to be given to the employee to help them accept their needs and capacities have changed.

> In many cases, denial in persons with HD is due to brain dysfunction. For example, when neurons die, feedback loops become disconnected so that information cannot travel from one part of the brain to another. As a consequence many people with HD suffer from lack of self awareness and don't recognise their disabilities. (Huntington's Society of Canada 1996)

Limitations on being able to drive a car, operate dangerous machinery or being trusted with previous responsibilities need to be approached sensitively. People with HD can be very impulsive and demand to see someone or something immediately and will not settle until their request has been fulfilled. As many people with HD are young and still physically fit and active they can be difficult to restrain if they wish to carry out a particular activity. Carers may need an emergency number for help and advice and occasionally mental health, social work and police assistance may be required.

Meeting new challenges as the disease progresses

The middle and late stages of HD can last for up to ten years. By the middle stages the person with HD can no longer work and has lost the ability to initiate any household chores or organise or plan the ordinary activities of daily living. However, they are physically capable of managing to carry out many tasks with encouragement and support. It is likely that memory will be a problem and the person may become short tempered over small issues. These symptoms are often reported to be more distressing to the carer than the physical symptoms. This is also the stage when many of the physical symptoms of the illness become obvious; involuntary movements can no longer be disguised, speech becomes less clear, swallowing becomes more problematic. The carer needs to be very organised and have an abundance of energy if they are to continue working and caring. The family should be given every emotional and practical support from the multidisciplinary team.

How the multidisciplinary team can support the HD family

The GP will often be the person the family goes to for help. GPs can:

- encourage referral to regional genetic services to enable the family to be given correct genetic information; many centres have contact with the voluntary organisations involved with HD or have their own nurse adviser who can have ongoing contact with the family

- develop their own knowledge of HD, testing procedures and specialist services available
- refer to a specialist, usually a psychiatrist or neurologist, who can give advice on medication to treat HD symptoms where necessary
- encourage family members to visit the surgery regularly to discuss their situation so that crises can be predicted
- discuss respite options with the carer and encourage them to consider this from an early stage in the disease
- support the carer if they have made the choice not to care at home any longer.

A number of other practitioners can also provide valuable input into families with HD. The *district nurse* in the primary care team can:

- help with bathing and provision of suitable bathing aids
- assess continence and assess the reason, e.g. urine infection; the inability to reach the toilet due to mobility problems, or inability to undo small clips and buttons
- advise on suitable clothing and, if necessary, appropriate aids with regular reassessment as the disease progresses
- advise the carer on skin care, giving of medication, bathing and lifting and handling.

Speech and language is a key area for therapy and can make a significant difference in terms of the continuation and quality of communication and management problems with eating and swallowing. A *speech and language therapist* can:

- educate the person with HD and the carer in regular exercises to maintain intelligible speech for as long as possible, reducing some of the frustration suffered
- assess swallowing and provide advice on the consistencies of food which could be causing a problem
- educate the person with HD and the carer about positioning during eating and drinking, how to achieve the correct consistency of food for safety, how to encourage the person with HD to eat slowly to prevent choking. All carers should have a knowledge of how to per-

form the Heimlich manoeuvre to dislodge material obstructing the airway.

People with HD can have an insatiable appetite but continue to lose weight. Maintaining body weight is extremely important to maintain optimum functioning and quality of life. A *dietician* can:

- give advice on how to increase the calorific value of food to give more calories per meal without increasing the volume of food, especially if swallowing is a problem
- advise the GP on suitable dietary supplements for prescription.

Physiotherapy advice is offered to:

- improve or maintain functional ability and promote safe mobility
- educate on regular exercises to achieve maximum mobility
- assess the need for aids to help with maintenance of safe mobility.

An *occupational therapist* can:

- perform home assessment and offer aids for the activities of daily living
- advise on major changes, e.g. a floor-level shower being installed
- assess and advise for suitable seating
- provide aids for safety e.g. smoking aid or community alarm
- provide information about room layout, design for dementia etc.

The *social worker* will work closely with other members of the team. Tasks will include:

- carrying out an assessment for the person and the carer on their needs
- introducing the idea of day centre/day activities, sitting services and respite and offer support in reviewing the options most acceptable to the person with HD and the carer; the social needs of the client need to be maintained and can be met by offering a befriending service or employment of a one-to-one carer in the same age range as the person with HD
- carrying out a benefit check to ensure the person with HD and the carer are receiving all the available benefits and refer welfare rights advice for employment, financial, or legal advice
- introducing and monitoring the care package and increasing care or introducing new services where necessary

- offering assistance and support to the person with HD and their carer. Should the person with HD require long-term care, especially if he/she is resisting and the carer is unable to cope, then specific counselling may be necessary. It is essential that the carer is supported appropriately and every effort should be made to find a care setting with experience of HD and with a philosophy of care which continues to maximise potential and promote individuality. Caring for the person with HD, in a residential setting, in a way which appropriately meets their physical and social needs is particularly challenging (see Chapter 13). This is likely to increase the cost of an appropriate residual place but is essential if the person's quality of life is to be maintained.

Planning and developing services for HD families

Many professionals in the fields of medicine, nursing, professions allied to medicine as well as social workers have a lack of specialist knowledge of HD but are required to provide advice and support to the HD family. This is often acknowledged by the professionals who turn to the advisory and genetic services for support. The situation is compounded by reduced training budgets in all professional areas.

Pressure on services means that speech therapy, physiotherapy and social activity programmes can be hard to access for the individual with HD. Provision of services across the country is inconsistent and patchy (HAS 1996).

Many agencies would be able to provide an excellent service to HD families if they had staff trained specifically to care for young people with a dementing illness. However, HD is further compounded by physical symptoms and genetic implications and additional training is required.

The care needs of HD families are very complex, and emotional as well as physical needs require attention. The carer struggles with the thought of their children developing the illness and how the child will cope with seeing their parent progress through the illness. In many other illnesses the adult children help with caring but with HD it can be difficult for adult children to offer support to their parents as they may be unable to watch the effects of HD because they fear they may develop HD themselves. In other instances there are no adult children to offer care for the parent.

The carer also has to cope with the loss of the future they had hoped for and, in many circumstances, the loss of financial security.

A nominated key worker/care manager with knowledge of HD, to coordinate all the specialist services and provide education to each specialist involved, is vital to provide quality care. Any significant information should be recorded in a mutually used communication folder, kept in the family home and discussed at regular meetings to ensure all the needs are being met. The poor coordination of services was highlighted in a recent report: 'There is a need for facilities to be developed to provide a service to the person with HD from early in the disease process until the end of life' (HAS 1996, p.50).

The person with HD requires care in an environment which is cheerful and includes young people, but which does not necessarily exclude the older people. The building should consider the physical disability which accompanies HD and the fact the many people with HD are in their 30s and 40s and may have young children. The care setting should accommodate the needs of children and encourage them to visit. The whole ambience of the care setting should be warm and welcoming as children who visit their parents in this setting may be 50 per cent at risk; may have had a positive test; or be in the early stages of the illness themselves. If the care facility meets the needs of the person with HD this will help relatives cope with their own status. As one of the symptoms of HD is the lack of ability to accept change, the care setting should offer day care, respite care and continuing care. The person with HD would start day care as soon as they accept it, closely followed by the introduction of respite care along with day care (which can be given as and when the person and their family wish). If it is then necessary to consider continuing care, the person with HD will not have to learn new routines or new faces at this late stage of their illness, with the added advantage that the care staff will also have known the person with HD whilst they were still able to express many of their likes and dislikes.

Respite facilities for the person with HD

Respite care can be difficult to find for reasons such as:

- the nursing home may not have registration for residents under 60
- the person with HD may not meet referral criteria, e.g. no behavioural problems
- financial cost for the family.

Services orientated to younger people with dementia may be much more appropriate than those for older people.

Continuing care setting for a person with HD

Although there are a few specialist units throughout the UK providing appropriate care, in Scotland there is only one residential home specifically offering specialist care for young people with HD. Transport and travel to this unit for many Scottish families is difficult and as a result they are forced to choose between specialist care for the person with HD and the difficulty in maintaining contact with them. To offer the best service to the HD family the multidisciplinary team needs to be involved throughout any period in residential care.

Experience has shown that a mix of general trained nurses and psychiatric trained nurses provide a good balance when caring for the HD resident. It is important to the family, especially to the individuals at risk, to feel there is a care centre with staff who are knowledgeable about HD and with a clear aim to provide the best quality of life possible. Facilities should be particularly sensitive to the needs of relative carers.

Case study: Margaret

Margaret is a 43-year-old lady with HD. She was 32 when she was told she had symptoms. Margaret is married with two children, Amy, 23, and Lorraine, 17. Amy has a son who is two years old. Margaret's husband has recently left her, Amy lives with her boyfriend and Lorraine lives at home with her mum.

Margaret has one brother aged 29 and a sister, Sarah. Sarah had taken the presymptomatic test six years ago, when direct gene testing was not available. She was shown to have only a 4 per cent chance of carrying the gene but has declined the offer of the new direct gene test.

Margaret tried to be as independent as possible; she had a home help for one hour every day and attended a day centre two days per week. Lorraine attended school nearby and came home everyday at lunch time to ensure her mum had all she needed for the next few hours until the school day ended. Lorraine then helped with making the dinner and washing up the dishes. Amy dealt with most of the other household needs, such as finance, shopping, repairs and dealings with the social work department.

After five years Margaret's physical condition and cognitive impairment had progressed to a point where a much more extensive home support system was needed following a community care assessment.

Margaret now requires help from her daughters, GP, occupational therapist, social worker, Huntington's adviser, speech therapist, day centre and a private care agency. All of these people provide almost 24-hour care for Margaret. Respite care is provided in a residential home which has a special interest in people with HD. This has progressed from one week every three months to two weeks in the residential home, six weeks in the community.

This intensive home support programme lasted for about a year, but Margaret now has a number of problems with swallowing and weight loss. She also smokes and this is creating a major fire risk to herself and to other tenants in the flats where she lives. At a case conference the options are discussed with Margaret, one being to consider long-term care in the unit she already attends for respite. It takes a while for Margaret and her family to come to terms with this but eventually everyone decides that it is the only solution for their situation and the whole family are given support during the transition.

One year on Margaret cannot walk independently but still has her outgoing personality and remains as independent as she can. She is now being carefully monitored and assisted for her swallowing problems and her weight loss but enjoys social occasions, being involved in her day-to-day care and seeing her family.

Margaret's daughter Lorraine is now in her own flat and working. She is considering having the test to find out if she carries the gene.

Amy is trying to fill the gap left by her mother going into care. She will not have the test for herself nor would she have the foetus tested if she was to become pregnant again.

The family, especially her daughters, visit Margaret regularly and are pleased that the residential unit encourages them to be involved in caring for her when they visit and in the life of the home.

This case study is based on a number of real-life situations as they progressed over time. Some people may be able to identify similarities to their own situations as many of the scenarios are common to HD families. All names have been changed to maintain confidentiality.

Positive developments in the care of the person with HD

In the UK, the voluntary organisations, Scottish Huntington's Association and the Huntington's Disease Association employ advisers providing a service in several areas. The advisory services are developed to meet the needs of HD families and provide education to both families and the professional and are solely funded by grants and fundraising. When health boards and social work authorities are planning the development of services they should consider funding for specialist voluntary organisations to provide specialist services. The role of the advisers cross both health and social work boundaries. Development of a UK wide advisory service has been hindered by lack of funds.

Internationally the approach to service provision differs from country to country. In Belgium, social workers are employed to provide an advisory service, whereas in Spain volunteers offer support and education to families through the voluntary organisations. Canada and America both have well-developed services for supporting families and also provide educational material for professionals and families. Through the Huntington's associations worldwide, information is shared and adapted for use in each country.

The International Huntington's Association (IHA) assists countries developing a HD organisation, facilitates the international sharing of new educational resources, encourages basic and clinical research and addresses ethical concerns.

In Scotland there is a grant-funded project which includes the development of an integrated care pathway for the person with HD based on recommendations of a multidisciplinary working group, which is expected to be in place by January 1998.

A report on the effectiveness of and the reasons for not complying with the pathway will be compiled and published. This is undoubtedly a major step in providing a more comprehensive service for HD families. Deviations noted in the pathway record are likely to be due to the lack of resources available in certain areas and a benefit of the project will be a documentation of the gap between recommendations and reality.

In August 1997, scientists from London, Germany and the United States reported a breakthrough in their research. The studies identify brain cell death as being caused by clumps of protein forming in the cell nucleus, leading to the progressive physical and mental symptoms associated with HD. Although it will be a lengthy process, there is growing hope that drugs can be found which target this process leading to more specific and effective treatment.

Families will continue to need active support from a wide range of health and social care agencies who need to work collectively and in partnership with the families involved to develop more coordinated and locally available services sensitised to the particular needs of those affected by Huntington's disease.

Further reading

Campbell, H., Hotchkiss, R., Bradshaw, N. and Porteous, M. (1998) 'Integrated care pathways'. *British Medical Journal 316*, 133-137.

CHAPTER 7

Learning Disabilities and Dementia

Sally-Ann Cooper

Introduction to learning disabilities

Learning disabilities (mental retardation) is the term used in the United King-dom to describe people whose intellectual ability is significantly lower than that of the average person, and who additionally do not learn/acquire the usual full range of adaptive/self-care skills. Onset of these difficulties occurs during the person's developmental phase (i.e. childhood) which distin-guishes between long-standing intellectual disabilities (learning disabilities) and intellectual disabilities acquired later in adult life (dementias). Intellec-tual ability is considered to be significantly lower than that of the average person if it is more than two standard deviations away from the mean, i.e. an intelligence quotient (IQ) of 70 points or less. If the IQ of the whole popula-tion was normally distributed, one would expect about 2 per cent of the population to fall within this category. However, there are a higher than expected number of births of people with severe and profound learning dis-abilities, due to the effects of genetic disorders and obstetric complications.

There are many causes of learning disabilities. In some cases, the learning disabilities are due to natural variation: not every person is the same, and some people are more or less able than others. Some people have learning disabilities due to particular disorders such as: genetic disorders (Down's syn-drome is an example of a chromosomal disorder; phenylketonuria is an example of a single gene disorder); brain injury (birth trauma; head injury in childhood); infective causes (e.g. following meningitis/encephalitis); ante-natal infections (e.g. maternal rubella); other antenatal complications (e.g. placental insufficiency, maternal alcoholism, intrapartum anoxia). Conse-quently, the population of people with learning disabilities is very varied. Some people are only delayed in their development; others have additional disabilities and in some cases multiple disabilities. A person with Down's syndrome, for example, may have hearing and visual impairments, cardiac defects, obesity, skin disorders and be prone to repeated respiratory infections, in addition to having learning disabilities. Another person with Down's syndrome may have delayed milestones (e.g. not walking or starting to talk until a much later age than usual), require special education as a child, and require some help with daily living and self-care skills when an adult, but otherwise be fit, healthy and psychologically well adjusted.

Although each person with learning disabilities is different and has differing needs, some experiences are shared. During childhood, their development is delayed (late in reaching milestones, or failing to reach some milestones such as walking, talking). There is usually a period of adjustment for the family of the child with the discovery that the child has learning disabilities. Such adjustment often takes time, with the family often moving through stages of shock, denial, anger and guilt before acceptance or in some cases rejection or overprotection of the child. This period of adjustment/ development of the family naturally also has an impact upon the development of the child with learning disabilities. Children with learning disabilities often require special education either in special schools or special classes in mainstream schools: this may set them apart from the average child. Adult life often revolves around the local learning disabilities day centre, special needs college courses or special supported work schemes/work cooperatives, rather than the usual work environment of the average adult. Even with the advent of community care and 'ordinary living' approaches many leisure activities are focused on the learning disabilities community, with special clubs, or activities and outings run by staff working for social services, private and voluntary organisations. The majority of adults with learning disabilities do not marry or have children. Despite enormous progress being made with the introduction of community care for people with learning disabilities, and the widespread popularisation of the principles of normalisation and social role valorisation, some people with learning disabilities are exposed to neglect, exploitation and abuse. Some people still see learning disabilities as a stigma. For all these reasons, the life experiences of people with learning disabilities often differ from that of the average person, as their expectations also differ from others. Social networks tend to be different: family networks in particular are primarily parents (until their death), and the maintenance of friendship networks are often dependent upon the support of others because of the practicalities of transportation and telephone calls.

Changing care needs of a person with learning disabilities

A person with learning disabilities is likely to have lifelong needs for additional care and support: this may range from 24-hour nursing care for those with profound learning disabilities and multiple physical disabilities to, at the other end of the spectrum, a few hours per week of support/home care or day care to help a person to live alone in their own home. However, the needs of a person with learning disabilities are not static, and do change. For some people, their need for additional care very slowly reduces, as through experience, training and practice, they gradually learn and acquire life skills and confidence. For other people, needs can increase. This may occur during discrete periods of time, for example when a person is unwell or undergoing a particularly stressful time, perhaps due to experiencing multiple life events, such as the death of a second parent and with that the loss of the family home. Alternatively, needs may change and increase on a more permanent basis. Some genetic disorders cause disabilities that are progressive, for example visual impairment due to retinitis pigmentosa, mobility impairment due to degenerative neurological disorders. The onset of dementia is an example of how the needs of a person with long-standing care needs may change due to additional psychiatric disorders.

Epidemiology of dementia

Dementia and Down's syndrome

People with learning disabilities due to Down's syndrome are particularly at risk of dementia (Holland and Oliver 1995; Oliver and Holland 1986). Neuropathological studies have demonstrated that by the age of 40 years, almost 100 per cent of people with Down's syndrome who die have the microscopic changes in the brain associated with Alzheimer's disease (tangles and plaques). However, clinical dementia does not appear to be this prevalent: a significant number of middle-aged and elderly people with Down's syndrome are alive and well with no signs of having dementia. It has proven difficult so far to explain this discrepancy between brain pathology and clinical well being/health. Research studies have examined people with Down's syndrome using the different approaches of repeated measures of adaptive behaviour, psychometric assessments, psychiatric assessment or neurological assessment. Due to these differing study methodologies, it is not possible to directly compare results from many of the studies. However, it appears that dementia (as opposed to brain pathology/microscopic changes of Alzheimer's disease) occurs in people with Down's syndrome at a rate of 2.0 per cent for the age group 30–39 years; 9.4 per cent for the group aged 40–49 years; 36.1 per cent for the group aged 50–59 years and 54.5 per cent for the group aged 60–69 years (Prasher 1995).

It is unclear exactly why dementia occurs commonly amongst young/middle-aged people with Down's syndrome. Theories have been proposed to account for this, including the implication of genetic material on chromosome 21: both superoxide dismutase and amyloid precursor protein are coded for on chromosome 21, and have been implicated as contributory to the dementing process. It has also been suggested that the role of apolipoprotein e in dementia is relevant, and there is a different distribution of this in people with Down's syndrome compared with the general population. The very high rates of dementia amongst people with Down's syndrome provides a model which may uncover important understandings that are of relevance to the whole population with dementia.

Although Down's syndrome is the commonest single genetic cause of learning disabilities, it accounts for only a minority of people with learning disabilities. About 20 per cent of adults with moderate–profound learning disabilities have Down's syndrome. The life span of people with Down's syndrome is increasing, but is not as long as that of people with learning disabilities of many other causes. Hence the proportion of people with Down's syndrome out of the total reduces, with increasing age cohorts. People with learning disabilities of other causes do not yet live as long as people from the general population, but their life span is also increasing (due in part to better care and lifestyles, and access to medical treatments that in the past were denied). Jacobson, Sutton and Janicki (1985) summarised this by stating that the people with learning disabilities who lived the longest were those who were female, had less severe learning disabilities, were ambulatory, did not have Down's syndrome and had remained living in the community. However, the high rates of dementia occurring in young and middle-aged people with Down's syndrome do have a significant impact on service demand as well as affecting the lives of individual people and their families/carers, which will increase as life span increases further.

Dementia and learning disabilities of causes other than Down's syndrome

The majority of people with learning disabilities do not have Down's syndrome. Dementia also occurs commonly amongst people with learning disabilities due to causes other than Down's syndrome (Cooper 1997a). Although the prevalence rates are not as high as they are for people with Down's syndrome, they are much higher than the prevalence rates which would be found in the general population of similar age. It is again difficult to directly compare the results of existing research studies, as they have used different methodologies, for example, different populations (hospital-based versus community-based populations), different methods of collecting information (analysing case notes versus psychiatric assessments of individuals and informant interviews) and differing diagnostic criteria. Three epidemiological studies were undertaken to determine the rate of dementia in people with learning disabilities (Cooper 1997a; Lund 1985; Moss and Patel 1993). These studies all provide comparable rates with dementia occurring in about 13 per cent of people with learning disabilities aged 50 years and over, and 22 per cent of people aged 65 years and over. This is about four times higher than one would expect from an age-matched general population.

People with learning disabilities are, of course, vulnerable to all the same risk factors for dementia as are the general population. Similar associations of dementia have been demonstrated for people with learning disabilities as for the general population, such as increasing age, increased number of additional physical disorders, more poorly controlled epilepsy; and protective factors, such as smoking (Cooper 1997a). Clearly though, in addition to these similarities, there must be additional factors which make people with learning disabilities more vulnerable to developing dementia. At this stage, it is only possible to speculate what these factors may be, as further research is required. Genetic factors may well be implicated. Alternatively, the dementia may be related to the 'brain damage' of many causes which is aetiological to the learning disabilities: head injury in the general population is known to increase the risk of a person later developing dementia, an extreme example of this being dementia pugilistica (boxer's dementia). Another possible explanation for the high prevalence rates is that dementia is detected at a much earlier stage when it occurs in people with learning disabilities, perhaps due to lack of brain 'reserve', i.e. a very small change affecting the brain can make a big difference to a person's abilities when he/she already has limited daily living and self-care skills. However, this latter explanation is unlikely, as work with people with Down's syndrome has shown that dementia tends to be detected during its later stages, and is difficult to detect in the early stages: it seems unlikely that the converse should be true for people with learning disabilities of other causes.

Clinical presentation of dementia

The changes that occur in dementia amongst people with learning disabilities are similar to those seen amongst the general population. However, due to the different lifestyles of people with learning disabilities compared with the average person, and the communication difficulties that are often present, the timing and nature of the first indication of possible dementia is often different. For the average person, he/she may become aware of some of the subtle cognitive changes at an early stage; for example, may complain of having a poor memory before others have noticed this. In some cases, the first warning of a problem may be a decline in a person's performance at work, which a supervisor/manager or colleague may notice: or the person him/herself may no longer feel able to keep up with work. A spouse or other significant person in his/her life may notice changes in the person's memory, judgement, thinking. However, these situations are less likely to arise for the person with learning disabilities. Communication problems may limit the person's ability to describe any changes he/she is aware of, and it may not be immediately obvious to carers if a person has memory problems if they have non-existent or limited verbal skills. Work at a learning disabilities day centre is unlikely to involve a high level of responsibility, so a small decline in performance may pass unnoticed. Unfortunately, many people with learning disabilities do not have a special one-to-one relationship with another person, once they have lost their parents (formal carers are often shared with several other people with learning disabilities), so again, early changes may pass undetected.

Case study 1: Mr A

Staff who are unaware of the early signs of dementia may miss significant small changes. For example, Mr A, a man in his early 50s, had attended a day centre regularly for the last ten years. He started to take someone else's coat every time he left the centre. The staff thought he was just getting more tired during the day because his residential carer had mentioned he was not sleeping so well. On a couple of occasions he had been found in a different part of the building after going to the toilet: he said he wanted to see what the builders were doing. Alterations were being made to the back of the centre and the staff thought that Mr A's confusion was partly explained by this as well as his sleeping pattern being disrupted.

People with learning disabilities have cognitive impairments as part of their underlying condition. Consequently, short tests of cognitive function that are often used with the general population are not applicable as 'one-off' screening instruments for this group of people (although they may be used to assess how a disorder, once established, is progressing). An example would be the Mini-Mental State Examination (Folstein, Folstein and McHugh 1975) where a score under 24 may seem to demonstrate an abnormality in someone drawn from the general population. However, someone with learning disabilities may score less than 24 on this test even though he/she is healthy and well. It would be difficult to use the test at all with someone with no verbal skills. The key factor in assessing the presence of dementia amongst people with learning disabilities is demonstrating that a change from the person's usual level of functioning/ability has taken place. This requires taking detailed information from a key informant in all cases, and never relying only on an interview with the person with learning disabilities him/herself. In practice, this can cause difficulties when parents are no longer available to consult, as paid carers often have knowledge of the person over only a short period of time, due to people changing residence (in some cases, unfortunately, because of their changing needs), and carers leaving posts through job changes, maternity leave, promotion or moving away. Such difficulties point to the need for detailed life history information and records being kept by the carer/key worker and regularly updated through the review process.

With careful assessment the usual symptoms of dementia can be seen. This includes impaired memory, for example forgetting where items are placed and which events were attended, compared with previous memory ability; forgetting names of people which used to be known; getting lost in previously familiar places; being unable to follow instructions that previously were easily followed (or only half completing tasks that used to be accomplished easily); no longer recognising familiar people. Impairments of other cognitive skills such as judgement and thinking also occur, for example mixing up day and night (getting up in the middle of the night insistent that it is time for work); loss of ability in reading or writing skills; loss of ability to budget or count change or handle money (compared with previous money skills); loss of specific self-care skills, such as shampooing hair, washing, shaving, dressing, shopping. In this context, loss of skills includes both an inability to do tasks previously completed, or requiring more verbal prompts and reminders to complete tasks. Other psychiatric symptoms may also occur as a result of dementia, such as depressive symptoms including irritability, apathy, loss of self-direction skills, reduced speech and social interaction, and changes in existing personality traits.

Psychotic symptoms commonly occur amongst people with learning disabilities and dementia. More than a quarter of the people examined in one study were found to have psychotic symptoms, with the most common type of symptoms being delusions of theft, other persecutory delusions and visual hallucinations of strangers in the house (Cooper 1997b). Other symptoms found to occur are change in sleep pattern, loss of concentration, worry, change in appetite and the onset of, or increase in levels of aggressive behaviour (Moss and Patel 1995; Cooper 1997c). A study of people with Down's syndrome who have dementia has also shown that non-cognitive psychiatric symptoms occur (Prasher 1995; Prasher and Filer 1995).

Case study 2: Ms W

Ms W is a 42-year-old woman with severe learning disabilities due to Down's syndrome who has always lived with her mother who is now aged 82. Her mother was concerned that Ms W had changed over the last six months. She would no longer tell her mother what she had done at the day centre when she came home and was irritable when asked about this. Sometimes she seemed muddled up about things and needed more prompting with her personal hygiene. Some days she didn't have her bag with her when she came home and didn't know where it was. Ms W's mother spoke with her key worker at the day centre who said that Ms W had recently chosen to stop some of her sessions, including current affairs and literacy skills. Ms W started to get up in the middle of the night, insistent that it was time to get ready for the day centre. This led to arguments between her and her mother, which was stressful for both of them. The community learning disabilities team undertook a full health assessment and social needs assessment. The psychiatrist diagnosed that Ms W had dementia and excluded any other psychiatric or physical causes that could have contributed to her changing behaviour. From the assessment, a care plan and a care package were designed to support Ms W and her mother in the wish they both expressed that Ms W would continue to live at home. The community learning disabilities nurse and care manager took the lead in implementing the care plan and in regularly reviewing the care package. It was unclear how long Ms W's elderly mother would be able to continue caring for her: one future alternative would be for Ms W to move to the private care home where she currently receives regular respite care, or a home providing 24-hour staffed support; a familiar environment preferred, to reduce disorientation.

Management of dementia

Health assessment

When it is first noticed that a person's needs are changing, or the person has new symptoms, it is important to undertake a comprehensive health assessment in order to accurately determine why. This must be done in a way that is sensitive to the anxieties and concerns of the individual and their relative/carer/advocate. Such an assessment is essential for three main reasons.

- The changes may be due to a treatable condition, which, with the appropriate remedies, may be reversed. There are several such conditions which either mimic dementia, or may be thought of as reversible dementias, e.g. depression, hypothyroidism, hearing/visual impairment, infections.

- If dementia is diagnosed, treating all other health problems that are additionally present may maximise a person's functional ability.

- Following a diagnosis of dementia, the individual and carer may be offered information and advice on support, management strategies and prognosis, so that sensible planning for the future is possible.

The comprehensive health assessment includes the following components.

1. It is essential to take a history from both the individual and an informant (ideally who has known the person long enough to describe the differences between how he/she is now compared with in the past). This history includes details of the changes noticed by the carer(s), specific questions about memory, other cognitive skills, and the full range of potential psychiatric symptoms of dementia and other psychiatric illnesses. Past psychiatric and medical illnesses and treatments are detailed, and specific medical information collected about any epilepsy and/or sensory impairments. Medication histories should be collected, and also details of medical and psychiatric illnesses amongst family members. A personal history and social history are also required, as is a developmental assessment. Questions should also be asked to review all bodily systems in order to detect previously undiagnosed medical illness.

2. A mental state examination is undertaken: this is largely conducted simultaneously with the history taking, and assesses appearance and behaviour, speech, affect and mood, thoughts, psychotic phenomena, cognition and insight.

3. A physical examination should be undertaken of all bodily systems, including sensory systems.

4. Special investigations will be required. This includes blood tests for full blood count, erythrocyte sedimentation rate, urea and electrolytes, liver function tests, blood glucose level, thyroid function tests, serum vitamin B12 and red cell folate, and syphilis serology. A urine sample should be sent for microscopy and culture to exclude infection, and a chest X-ray taken. Further investigations may be indicated, depending upon the results from the history, mental state and physical assessments. Neuroimaging studies, such as computerised tomography (CT) scans, are often unhelpful (unless there is a previous scan with which a comparison can be made) as such scans are often abnormal due to long-standing disorders. CT scans may be indicated, however, in particular circumstances to exclude other organic pathologies such as hydrocephalus (which is particularly associated with tuberous sclerosis) or a space-occupying lesion (when there are focal signs on examination, or symptoms of raised intercranial pressure).

When these four stages of the assessment have been completed, it is usually possible to diagnose (or exclude) dementia with confidence.

Multidisciplinary/multiagency care planning

The further management of dementia depends upon the person's individual circumstances, but is likely to require multidisciplinary/multiagency input to devise a care plan to address the following issues:

1. Correction of any disorders/difficulties that have been identified, such as treatment of anaemia, urine infection or other physical illness; referral for any hospital treatments required; prescription for new glasses or hearing aid; dental treatment; replacement of poorly fitting shoes.

2. Information for carer and individual. This involves explanations about dementia, the fact that the person may still have many quality years of life ahead of him/her, but that the condition is progressive. It is important to explain that the loss of skills is not because the person is not trying, but that he/she is no longer able, and that expectations of carers have to be tailored to meet changing needs and capacity. The carer may wish to be put in contact with local voluntary organisations and dementia societies. It may be appropriate to discuss the types of services that are available for future needs. In some cases, it may, sadly, be necessary to discuss whether the person's current home is likely to meet their needs in the near and distant future, or whether a change of residence will be necessary; and if so, when and how this should be handled. It is unlikely that

a carer could assimilate all of this information in one appointment, unless they are already very well informed. It is important to understand the high emotional impact of such information. Consequently, this is likely to involve planned sessions with the psychiatrist, nurse, psychologist or social worker/care manager to work through these issues. The length of time required for this process will depend upon the particular circumstances of the individual and the carer/support network. Written information may also be helpful.

3. Advice on minimising cognitive symptoms of dementia. Some of the principles of reality orientation can be applied to work with people with learning disabilities and dementia. This may include structuring the day so that sequences of events occur in the same order/at the same time every day. Reminding the person about the plan of activities for the day, prompting him/her repeatedly as to what happens when, and which part of the day it is now, is helpful. Using a pictorial daily planner of the day's events, helping the person to put a tick beside each event/meal once it is over and then encouraging the person to use the planner to check what happens next may be useful. Other simple steps are to clearly label rooms to help the person in finding his/her way around at home (e.g. a picture of a WC on the door of the WC, a picture of a bed on the bedroom door). The use of written lists and written diaries is less likely to be helpful for people who cannot read or write. A life-story book of photographs of significant people and places may be a useful way to facilitate reminiscence (and provides useful information for formal carers). There may be a role for specific pharmacotherapy to improve cognitive function.

4. Non-cognitive symptoms of dementia may require specific treatment. Such symptoms may cause more distress to the individual and carer than do the cognitive symptoms. When agitation is a problem, pharmacotherapy is sometimes effective, or relaxation techniques including massage, aromatherapy, soft music, use of Snoezelen rooms (multisensory stimulation rooms – see Chapter 13). Psychotic symptoms should be treated with antipsychotic drugs and reassurance and explanation to the individual and carer. If aggression occurs, the appropriate management will depend upon detailed assessment of the cause: it may for example, be due to psychotic symptoms or due to anxiety. Alternatively, it might be a 'catastrophic reaction' to demands being made of the individual which exceed his/her ability (which may then be remedied by advice to the carer on simplifying instructions and requests). The ag-

gression might alternatively be a symptom of the relative's/carer's own stress and difficulty in coping with a changing situation and inability to set clear boundaries. Such behaviour will require assessment, from which the appropriate management plan and support systems can be devised.

5. Provision of occupation, recreation and daily care. The amount of additional care that the person requires, for example for washing, dressing and feeding, will change as the illness progresses, and so requires continual review by the carer together with the social worker/care manager. The assessment of the individual's needs will be the basis from which the care package is devised, but this will require regular review. The provision of recreation and occupation is an important component of the care package, and may involve, for example, attendance at a day centre, or one-to-one time with a care worker. Some day centres can be noisy and busy leading to distress and anxiety for some individuals. With sensitivity, staff can do much to create a calmer and less hectic environment, but one which still provides interest, comfort, stimulation and enjoyment.

6. Support for carers. Each of the above areas should include the provision of support for carers. Caring for a loved family member with dementia, particularly when this person is the carer's child (most people with learning disabilities living with family are cared for by parents) is stressful, and includes many anxieties about the future. Emotional support through listening to the parents' concerns and trying to empathise (putting yourself in the parent's shoes) can be helpful, as can providing information (although the pace of this needs to vary for different people). Practical support is also essential, and will require the assessment of needs to include the circumstances and wishes of the parent(s) as well as the person with learning disabilities, for example provision of home carers or respite care. Such care packages require continual review as needs change. If parents no longer feel able to care for their son or daughter at home, or feel that their care would be better provided elsewhere, they may need help to come to terms with a move to residential care and with the practicalities of initiating such a move. Voluntary organisations play an important role in supporting carers in addition to the roles of health and social services and the private sector. Formal carers may also need considerable support from their managers, the multidisciplinary team and appropriate community support staff.

The best outcome for the individual with dementia is likely to be achieved in each of these areas when staff working in different disciplines and agencies collaborate effectively, and work to a shared action plan with agreed objectives and goals. The person's immediate carer/relative is the key ingredient in the implementation of support and management strategies, and so the provision of adequate explanation and support to the carer/relative is essential if the care plan is to be effective.

Future services and challenges in service provision

In the past it was unusual for people with learning disabilities to live into middle age. This has now changed due to access to medical treatments (e.g. antibiotics for chest infections, cardiac surgery for congenital heart defects) and better quality lifestyles and care. Learning disabilities services in the past were services for children and young adults which focused on learning, skill acquisition and development, increasing independence, encouraging choices, decision making, autonomy. These approaches remain an important component of learning disabilities services but are, however, less helpful when managing and supporting a person with dementia. For a person with dementia, maintaining skills but coming to terms with losses is a more appropriate focus than trying to learn new skills, though it is always important to maximise potential. People with learning disabilities aged 40 years and over now outnumber children with learning disabilities: consequently, learning disabilities services are required for a large number of adults. Dementia is common amongst people with learning disabilities, and will become more prevalent as life span continues to increase. However, learning disabilities services in many areas have not yet faced the challenge of meeting the needs of this group (Cooper 1997c).

A further change is that in the past, learning disabilities services were focused on hospital care, attempting to provide for all health and social care aspects of a person's life. This has changed with the move to community care provided in a variety of small homes and supported housing with social services taking the lead in social care. This raises the issue of care for people in the terminal stages of dementia, where social care providers are still developing their skills but nursing care in hospital is not now available. This issue reflects the youth of many community services which should improve with time, experience and multiagency cooperation and sharing of skills.

One must question whether the needs of people with learning disabilities and dementia are best met by specialist learning disabilities services, or by general services for people with dementia. Many of the health and social services, private and voluntary services provided in this country for people with dementia are particularly aimed at older people (as dementia occurs in many more elderly people than it does in younger people). This can cause difficulties for younger users of these services: reminiscence groups for example may not be able to span the generations. The younger person with learning disabilities has additional difficulties in using these services: his/her life experiences are likely to have been substantially different from a person of similar age from the general population. He/she may have lived for a large part of his/her life in an institution, never had paid employment, attended a day centre, and never married or had children. This may lead to the person with learning disabilities having difficulty in integrating into the group.

This presents a dilemma. In the United Kingdom, the health component of the person's care is often best provided by the specialist learning disabilities psychiatric, nursing and therapy services, but flexible and collaborative working with the general adult or old age psychiatrist services may be required. However, the social component of the person's care package is less easy to 'prescribe'. Elderly people with dementia outnumber younger people with dementia, for whom it is therefore more of a challenge to develop appropriate services. Younger people with dementia outnumber younger people with learning disabilities and dementia, and hence this latter group are less likely to be the target of dementia services. Equally, however, learning disabilities services are still developing the skills and knowledge to provide for this group. The answer to this dilemma lies in collaboration between agencies with users and carers. Drawing upon the experience and knowledge of learning disabilities services, social services for elderly people and people with dementia and private and voluntary organisations such as Age Concern, Alzheimer's Disease Society and Alzheimer Scotland – Action on Dementia, will result in local services which are sensitive to the needs of the local population.

CHAPTER 8

Alcohol-Related Brain Impairment

Simon Crowe

Introduction

Alcohol is the second most widely used and the most widely abused drug known to man. Written reports of the use of wine, beer and other intoxicants date back at least as far as 3000 BC, and the existence of intoxicants has been noted in numerous preliterate cultures and even in animals in the wild. However, despite our long history and experience of alcohol it remains a massive social problem.

Measured in terms of accidents, lost productivity, crime, death or damaged health, the combined social costs of problem drinking in the United States were estimated for 1980 to exceed $89 billion annually. The cost in broken homes, wasted lives, loss to society and human misery is beyond calculation (Jaffe 1985).

This chapter surveys the effects of alcohol abuse from a pharmacological, neurological, neuropsychological and public health perspective with a view to answering a number of crucial questions: What happens when we drink? What happens when we drink too much? What conditions occur as a consequence of alcohol abuse? Is there recovery from chronic alcohol-related brain impairment? What are the implications of the deficits associated with alcohol abuse for the provision of services and support?

What happens when we drink?

Alcohol is a reversible central nervous system (CNS) depressant, but a transient stimulant at low doses leading to the familiar release from anxiety and inhibition associated with drinking. After ingestion, it is absorbed through the stomach and intestines and from these sites is distributed throughout the body in proportion to the dose that has been ingested. About 95 per cent of the alcohol taken in is metabolised by the enzyme alcohol dehydrogenase which occurs mainly in the liver. The remaining 5 per cent is excreted largely unchanged through the lungs. This latter feature has made it possible for the development of alcohol breath testing, a very effective means of combating the problem of drink driving.

As the levels of ethanol exposure increase, more systems of the body become compromised. The most noticeable of these is the impairment of motor coordination. The slurring, poor coordination and stumbling gait associated with alcohol occur as a consequence of its effect on the cerebellum (the 'small brain' located at the back and to the bottom of the cerebrum or 'large brain'). Driving skill is impaired at relatively low doses, beginning at a blood alcohol concentration of 0.03 per cent but becoming much more marked by 0.08 per cent.

Although, as discussed later, alcohol can be quite a devastating neurotoxin (a substance that is capable of poisoning nerves), in moderation it has quite the opposite effect. Several recent reports have noted that alcohol in small doses may reduce the risk of coronary artery disease. The mechanism of this effect is reported to be that alcohol acts to increase levels of high-density lipoprotein (a chemical which contains both fat and protein and reduces damage to arteries) in blood with a proportionate decrease in low-density lipoprotein (a chemical which increases damage to arteries). This cardioprotective effect however is lost if the individual also smokes cigarettes (Julien 1995).

What happens when we drink too much?

The insult to the body and most particularly to the nervous system caused by alcohol comes about as a consequence of two separate but nonetheless associated processes. These are the neurotoxic effect of alcohol (or more specifically the breakdown product of alcohol, acetaldehyde), and the vitamin deficiency associated with alcoholism.

In pharmacological terms, alcohol is considered to be a relatively weak agent. This label has been awarded because it requires a considerable amount of alcohol to be ingested to cause its pharmacological effect. In comparison with other recreational drugs such as marijuana or LSD the doses required to achieve an effect with alcohol are many thousands of times larger. As such it seems unlikely that there are specific biochemical receptors on cells for alcohol. It is more likely that alcohol dissolves through the membranes of the nerve cells to achieve its effect.

Numerous candidates have been put forward to characterise the neuro-transmitter system implicated in alcohol's effect on the brain. These include serotonin, acetylcholine or glutamate (all neurotransmitters of the brain). At present glutamate is considered to be the most likely candidate, particularly by virtue of its action on N-methyl-D-aspartate (NMDA) receptors (specific sites which bind a particular neurotransmitter). For an agent that we think we know so well, it is surprising how much we do not know about the mechanism, or site of action of alcohol in the body.

The problem of alcohol abuse emerges because of the nature of alcohol as a product. It is not a whole food, and anyone who substitutes alcohol for a balanced diet is creating a situation in which they are relying on the alcohol for all of their nutritional requirements. Alcohol is generally described as containing 'empty calories'. Six hundred millilitres of 86 per cent proof spirit has the caloric value of 1500 k/cal, yet a bottle of Scotch contains no vitamins or amino acids. Long-term ingestion to excess leads to the emergence of malnutrition and vitamin deficiency. The vitamins that are deficient are mostly of the B group which includes thiamine (vitamin B1), riboflavin (vitamin B2), niacin (vitamin B3), pyridoxine (vitamin B6), folate and vitamin B12. There are also deficiencies in trace elements and other essential constituents including carnitine, vitamin A, zinc, magnesium and phosphate.

What conditions occur as a consequence of alcohol abuse?

As noted already, alcohol has an effect on almost every system in the body. As a consequence the medical problems associated with alcoholism occur in a variety of different systems and with a variety of effects. These are now reviewed system by system (Mackay 1992).

The gut and viscera

Alcoholism causes numerous disturbances of the gut. These include erosion of the lining of the stomach which is responsible for the nausea associated with the 'morning after'. It also produces liver disease. This occurs in a staged manner such that the more marked the abuse, the more marked is the pathology of the liver. The first stage is the accumulation of fat in the cells of the liver (so called fatty liver). This is followed by inflammation of the liver (alcoholic hepatitis). By this time the liver has begun to enlarge considerably and the skin may be jaundiced (yellowing of the skin due to the excretion of bile being blocked). As the level of drinking continues damage is exacerbated, scarring the liver (cirrhosis of the liver) leading finally to permanent liver failure. The development of these changes is usually quite slow, sometimes requiring more than 10 to 20 years of heavy drinking to produce the final pathology. The pancreas (responsible for the production of insulin) is also susceptible to alcohol-related change. This results in pathological changes in the organ and progressive destruction of its secretory function.

The cardio-vascular system

High blood pressure and cardiac failure are common effects of alcoholism, and as the level of drinking progresses, there is cardiac enlargement.

The skeleton and musculature

Osteoporosis (increased brittleness and loss of bone mass) is common amongst alcoholics resulting in a high incidence of bone fractures. There may also be muscle damage with loss of muscle bulk and bone marrow changes leading to deficits in blood clotting and anaemia. Alcohol has also been implicated in the emergence of cancers of the mouth and pharynx.

The reproductive system

Alcoholism can result in decreased levels of testosterone (a male sex hormone) and increased oestrogen (a female sex hormone), so that a male alcoholic often experiences a loss of sex drive and impotence. The hormonal changes can also lead to feminisation of the male presenting as the development of breast tissue. Alcohol consumed by pregnant women crosses the placenta.

The nervous system

The effects of alcohol on the nervous system can be divided into acute, semi-permanent and chronic effects.

ACUTE EFFECT OF INTOXICATION

The acute effects of alcohol begin with excitement and end with stupor or coma. In the early stages of intoxication, exhilaration and loss of inhibition occur. As consumption continues, a number of changes can be noted. These include: a decreased sensitivity to fine touch, a decrease in judgement and diminution of concentration and memory.

SEMI-PERMANENT EFFECTS

The semi-permanent effects of prolonged, frequent and excessive alcohol consumption include tolerance, dependence and problems associated with withdrawal. Tolerance is a condition in which the individual is relatively unaffected by a dose of alcohol that would be intoxicating for a social drinker. Clearly, the neurotoxic effect of alcohol remains unchanged as a consequence of the development of tolerance and as a result the individual is capable of taking in ever larger doses of the drug without the biological alarm signals of toxicity. As the brain adapts to ever larger doses of the drug, the individual becomes dependent upon alcohol to maintain his or her behavioural and emotional stability. Two interesting phenomena also may occur at about this stage. These include blackouts and idiosyncratic intoxication. Blackouts are periods of loss of memory for current events, which, according to the reports of colleagues or friends present at the time, were not associated with any unusual behavioural symptoms. They are associated with the severity of alcohol dependence, and are also more common in instances of a rapid increase in the blood alcohol concentration. Idiosyncratic or pathological intoxication is a situation in which an individual becomes quite drunk on what would ordinarily appear to be only a mild dose of alcohol. The problem often occurs in people with pre-existing brain injury.

The conditions associated with alcohol withdrawal are determined by the level of abuse. The most common symptoms and the times when they occur after withdrawal are: tremors (shaking of the body: 3–12 hours), hallucinosis (seeing things which are not there, for example pink elephants: 3–12 hours), seizures (so-called rum fits: 12–48 hours), delirium tremens (all three of these in association with agitation, confusion and sleep disorder: 3–4 days).

CHRONIC EFFECTS

The chronic effects of alcoholism include: cerebellar atrophy, peripheral neuropathy, hepatic encephalopathy, Wernicke's encephalopathy and Korsakoff's amnesic syndrome. These are described briefly as follows:

- Cerebellar atrophy manifests as disturbances of gait in the form of a wide-based gait in association with poor coordination of the movements of the legs. Interestingly, the changes to the cerebellum as a consequence of alcoholism are quite specific and it appears that only the anterior and superior parts of the cerebellum are affected by the drug.

- Peripheral neuropathy (nerve disease other than in the CNS) is a disturbance of the sensory functioning of the extremities, particularly of the feet. The impact of this sensory loss begins with the absence of the reflexes of the ankles, and can progress to more marked sensory abnormalities including numbness and pins and needles through to pain or burning sensations of the feet.

- Hepatic encephalopathy (disease of the brain caused by liver dysfunction) is a condition associated with the disorders of liver function discussed above. One of the roles of the liver is to detoxify the blood stream. As liver functioning becomes more compromised this ability diminishes resulting in increased levels of toxins in the blood. The principal neurotoxic substance in blood is ammonia (Butterworth 1995). The build up of this toxin can lead to marked disturbances of neurological function including cognitive and motor dysfunction, coma and death.

- Wernicke's encephalopathy (WE) is an acute neurological illness caused by severe deficiency of the vitamin thiamine (vitamin B1). It is acute in onset and is characterised by the classic triad of symptoms: eye signs, disorders of the control of the direction and coordination of the movements of the eyes including nystagmus, and abducens and conjugate gaze palsies (96%); ataxia of gait (77%) and a global confusional state (56%) (Victor, Adams and Collins 1989). Whilst thiamine deficiency is usually due to alcoholism, it is not the only cause and cases of WE attributable to anorexia nervosa, and to disorders associated with high levels of vomiting (e.g. hyperemesis gravidarum; severe vomiting during pregnancy) have also been noted. Alcoholism is responsible for the marked levels of thiamine deficiency because, as noted above, individuals who abuse alcohol have a tendency to be in a state of relatively poor nutrition. This leads to the replacement of food by drink, decreased absorption of thiamine and decreased storage and use of thiamine by the liver. WE can be reversed by the application of a 50–100mg dose of thiamine daily. WE is a medical emergency and if left unaided will result in coma and death.

- Korsakoff's amnesic syndrome is now generally considered to be the psychiatric manifestation of Wernicke's encephalopathy. Nowadays in recognition of this association, the common terminology Wernicke/Korsakoff syndrome (WKS) is used to describe both the acute and chronic effects of the condition. The characteristic amnesic syndrome of WKS shows a number of common features. These include an almost complete inability to learn new material, a normal short-term memory (for example the individual is able to repeat a telephone number immediately after looking it up in the telephone book), a retrograde amnesia with a temporal gradient (the individual is not capable of remembering events in his or her past life particularly for the period immediately preceding the emergence of the amnesia). The recall of events tends to be improved by direct questioning. There is generally preservation of early established skills and habits, for example language, gesture, well-practised skills and there also tends to be decreased initiative and spontaneity, together with blunting of affect. One of the fascinating features of the WKS is the tendency towards confabulation. This is defined as the tendency of the patient to produce erroneous material on being questioned about the past. This behaviour is more common in the early stages of the disorder and its emergence may be inversely related to insight into the condition. There are two types of confabulation (Berlyne 1972): momentary confabulation, in which in response to questions about his/her past the individual produces autobiographical material often of a habitual nature, and fantastic confabulation which is much less common and in which the individual produces material of a grandiose theme often arising spontaneously and frequently repeated. The material bears no relation to the individual's prior experience. The latter is probably due to impaired frontal lobe function, is commonly associated with an inability to inhibit incorrect responses, and is probably due to faulty self-monitoring.

- The well-fed alcoholic: though WKS is associated with the thiamine deficiency (Victor, Adams and Collins 1989) there are also alcoholics without WKS who have residual cognitive problems. These deficits are considered to be the neurotoxic effects of alcohol before the emergence of the WKS. Certainly in detoxified non-WKS alcoholics we can see residual deficits in those tests usually described as 'frontal' tests. Walsh (1994) has suggested that these features are due to the neurotoxicity of alcohol on the frontal lobes. Overall these individuals seem to have difficulty in developing new ideas and using the knowledge that they already have to apply it to new problems. As a consequence of this, they have a lot of difficulty in changing their behaviours and responding to new opportunities and possibilities. One aspect of this pattern of behaviour which is most worrying is the inability of these people to deal with the new generation of information technology such as automatic teller machines or voicemail telephone answering. Such changes often make it virtually impossible for these individuals to cope with the world with which they are now confronted.

How does alcohol abuse interfere with cognitive functioning?

A number of models of alcohol-related brain impairment (ARBI) have been proposed (Evert and Oscar-Berman 1995). These include the following.

- *The right hemisphere hypothesis.* This argues that alcoholics have specific dysfunction of the right hemisphere in comparison to other brain regions. To date studies using neuropsychological, electroencephalography (EEG) or computerised tomography (CT) scanning data have provided no support for the hypothesis.

- *The frontal system hypothesis.* Problems with problem solving, visual scanning, learning capacity and emotional arousal are commonly observed in alcoholics so that it has been argued that they may have frontal lobe deficits. It is currently argued that these deficits are not solely ascribable to frontal lesions but may be related to lesions spread throughout the brain. It is likely that the features are due to generalised deficits in higher level functioning. Although many can be ascribed to the frontal lobe damage this is not so invariably.

- *Abnormal ageing hypotheses.* The ageing hypotheses postulate that chronic alcohol abuse actually modifies the organism in such a way as to alter the biological mechanisms which mediate the process of normal ageing. This hypothesis has two forms, namely the premature ageing hypothesis and the accelerated ageing hypothesis. The accelerated ageing hypothesis contends that alcoholism is accompanied by the precocious onset of neuroanatomical changes typically associated with advancing age, whilst the increased vulnerability hypothesis contends that as the individual ages he/she becomes more prone to the neurodestructive effects of alcohol. Despite the attractiveness of these hypotheses there are no data as yet to support them (Evert and Oscar-Berman 1995).

- *The continuity hypothesis.* This hypothesis contends that there is a continuum of impairment associated with alcohol excess such that the more and the longer you drink the more likely it will be to cause brain impairment. Though intuitively appealing this hypothesis also has little support from the available data. Whilst there is a correlation between the level of abuse and level of impairment they are not necessarily interrelated and there are numerous individuals who show marked impairment (with only moderate levels of abuse) as well as those with profound drinking histories who display little if any deficit.

- *Possible acquired limitations in information processing.* This hypothesis contends that there is an intrinsic deficit in the way that information is processed by heavy drinkers. The argument is that poor motivation and poor use of strategies and their generalisation to a variety of situations may be the basis of poor test performance. As yet little data have been gathered to test this and there are no specific definitions as to what processes are compromised and how this could have happened.

In short, the explanatory models of ARBI are still in an imperfect state, and the trend in the literature at the moment is to approach the phenomena in a cognitive neuropsychological manner by attempting to find specific changes attributable to the effects of alcohol and explaining these on the basis of both neuroanatomical and cognitive evidence.

Is there recovery from ARBI?

This question presents as one of the most heart-rending and vexing questions in this area. The answer unfortunately is that no one knows. Certainly at the more extreme end of the spectrum, individuals with the WKS are relatively stable in terms of their cognitive deficits and as far as it has been possible to track these individuals (Victor, Adams and Collins 1989) there seems to be little long-term change in their cognitive functions. A group in which the findings are more encouraging are individuals who feature the dysexecutive syndrome associated with alcoholism, i.e. the non-WKS alcoholics. A number of recent studies (Drake *et al.* 1995) suggest that long-term follow up of non-WKS alcohol abusers provides evidence of restitution of function following abstinence. This indicates that there may well be scope for recovery or adaptation in these individuals who stop drinking.

What are the implications of the deficits associated with alcohol abuse to the provision of services and support?

As we have already noted, heavy alcohol consumption results in increasing risk of cognitive impairment, particularly in terms of executive functioning. Unlike other types of acquired brain damage such as traumatic brain injury or stroke, the changes associated with ARBI range from early changes resulting in decreasing cognitive flexibility and poor problem solving, through to the marked deficits in orientation, memory and independent functioning characteristic of the WKS.

In association with the multisystem injury associated with alcohol abuse, there are a number of additional barriers to effective service delivery. These include the following.

- In the early to intermediate stages of this spectrum of impairment, these individuals appear to be functioning quite normally. This can result in unrealistic expectations being placed on them, and when they do not carry them out, they are often labelled as uncooperative, unmotivated, difficult or just plain bloody minded.

- There is a stigma associated with alcohol abuse in so far as it is often considered to be a 'self-inflicted' injury. This results in a tendency to hide the problem on behalf of the individual and his or her family, preventing effective advocation on behalf of the individual.

- Many services and workers are inflexible in their philosophical belief that individuals are responsible for their actions and are able to make well-informed decisions for themselves. This places individuals who are not capable of this process due to their brain injury in a very precarious position.

- In Australia at least, eligibility criteria for service provision are often disability specific, and rarely if ever include alcohol-related brain impairment in their terms of reference.

- Individuals with ARBI are characterised by their inability to change or to deal with change. Insight-oriented approaches to achieving community integration fail. As these individuals cannot be changed the implication of service delivery to them means that the situation in which they exist must change to meet them. These are a group of individuals who are living by habit. The only approach to improvement must be by changing the environment which produces those habits.

Alcohol Related Brain Injury Assessment and Support Service

In response to the lack of any concerted approach to the issues of assessment and management of alcohol-related brain impairment, the Alcohol Related Brain Injury Assessment and Support Service (ARBIAS) was formed in

January 1989. The aim of ARBIAS was to redress the lack of services and support for people with ARBI in Victoria.

Victoria is the second most populous state of Australia with a population of 4,244,221 people as assessed by the 1991 census. Studies from several countries have shown that the neuropathology of WKS occurs with a prevalence of approximately 1 per cent to 3 per cent in post mortem studies (Thomson *et al.*1988). A prospective random survey of the incidence of Wernicke-Korsakoff neuropathology conducted in Sydney, New South Wales reported a prevalence of 2.2 per cent in the general population (Harper *et al.* 1989). In a more recent study, Harper and his group have noted that since the introduction of the fortification of flour with thiamine in Australia, the level fell to 1.1 per cent in a community sample. Whilst this figure indicates that fortification appears to be working, a sizeable number of individuals continue to suffer from WKS. Although precise figures are not available for Victoria, there seems no reason to assume that these epidemiological data do not apply to it. On the basis of Harper's most recent figure, then Victoria probably has around 47,000 individual cases of WKS.

If ARBI is the early stage of the WKS, and there are suggestions that it is a continuum (Lishman 1990), then the prevalence of WKS would indicate a high level of the early stages of the disease in the community. A recent stratified random sample study of drug use in Newcastle, New South Wales (Hancock *et al.* 1992) has indicated that 15.2 per cent of the males and 7.9 per cent of the females sampled were drinking hazardously (i.e. more than 28 standard drinks per week for males, more than 14 for females; National Health and Medical Research Council 1987), indicating that the problem potentially poses a massive public health threat. On the basis of these figures ARBIAS estimated that its population of interest may be as large as 500,000 individuals. Current UK government recommendations are a daily limit of no more than 3–4 units for men and 2–3 units for women with at least two alcohol-free days per week.

As its first order of business, ARBIAS investigated what the needs were for this group of clients and what the available services were. The findings were clear – there were no services in Victoria.

The needs identified by ARBIAS were:-

1. Assessment. If neuropsychological and neurological assessment were available, it would enable appropriate case planning and support for individuals and their carers.

2. Community awareness. If families understood the nature and implications of ARBI, and support was available, it is likely that many people would be able to remain in their own homes without significant institutionalisation.

3. Education, training and consultation. Part of the problem for this client group was that workers in government, non-government and residential services did not understand the nature of the disability, nor had the skills necessary to work effectively with this client group. More knowledge and dissemination of that knowledge would be crucial to ensure effective and appropriate care.

4. Long-term accommodation with support. The disability arising from ARBI results in an inability to cope with change due to the loss of the ability to plan and organise, or to learn new skills. If people were given the necessary specialised support to address their disability and to settle into secure, stable accommodation, they could become functioning and contributing members of the community.

In the years from inception to the present, ARBIAS has developed a unique model of service delivery for our client base. Activity now centres around four principal areas: the assessment unit, the case management service, the alcohol-free boarding house and the recreation project.

The assessment unit

The assessment unit provides three principal services:

1. a preliminary neurological examination which identifies any physical evidence of ARBI

2. access to further neurological investigations including magnetic resonance imaging, computerised tomography, electroencephalography or blood tests if indicated through a local publicly funded hospital

3. a full neuropsychological examination. This can identify the nature of the changes in cognitive function and the implications of these in terms of day-to-day functioning and prospects for rehabilitation.

The assessment process serves a number of useful purposes and addresses questions as diverse as:

• What are the problems an individual faces in independent living?

• Will he/she be able to return to work?

• Are there behavioural problems and how can these be managed?

- What type of accommodation and what level of supervision will be required?
- Can a strategic manipulation of either the environment or the individual's response to it be made to improve the level, duration and quality of independent functioning?

Arising from the assessment a management plan is developed including:

- feedback to the client as to his/her strengths and weaknesses
- detailed information to the case manager about the nature of the client's problems
- a review of how these problems will impact upon the client's day-to-day functioning in his/her normal environment
- provision of a strategy and plan for dealing with these problems for both the client and the case manager
- a realistic appraisal of what the individual can expect in terms of future recovery and level of disability.

The unit assessed 312 new clients from 1 July 1996 to 30 June 1997. Most came from public hospitals, GPs, community health centres or welfare organisations or as a consequence of the clients referring themselves. The demographic profile of the usual client referred to the service features a male aged from 31 to 65 years, likely to be non-aboriginal, unlikely to be in an ongoing relationship, likely to have completed some secondary education, likely to have worked previously at least at an unskilled manual level and unlikely to be employed currently and probably on welfare support. The levels of abuse and levels of brain impairment in the client base indicates that the clients abuse only alcohol and that nearly 90 per cent feature some level of brain impairment as a consequence of that abuse.

One figure that it is not possible to include here is the number of individuals who have not been evaluated and treated. As noted from estimates of the number of potential users of the service, many individuals go unrecognised and untreated by any service. The likelihood that such a population does exist is clearly illustrated by the observation in an autopsy study that though 1.1 per cent of the general population featured the neuropathological changes of WKS, this was rarely reported in life (Harper *et al.* 1989). Clearly many people are struggling with these problems without any help or service provision.

The case management service

The case management service developed by ARBIAS has proven to be one of our most effective means of aiding our client group. The service is founded on the philosophy that 'small things matter'. This translates into a programme of case management within which:

- the needs of the client take first priority
- once the individual becomes a client of ARBIAS the relationship does not end until a more appropriate service network becomes available
- response time is crucial: a small problem becomes a big problem in the time that it takes to respond to the initial phone call
- working with people with cognitive impairment is a slow process, and everything must be undertaken one slow and faltering step at a time
- behaviour and particularly challenging behaviour is a form of communication and every communication has a meaning and a reason.

Via the intervention of a flexible outreach case management system it has been possible to maintain many clients in the community with only a moderate level of ongoing support. From 1 July 1996 to 30 June 1997 the unit case managed 562 individual clients and a total of 5976 client contact hours were recorded. This approach is not just good for the clients, it represents a cheaper, more humane and ultimately more cost-effective means of management for a group of chronically disabled individuals living in the community.

The alcohol-free boarding house

The alcohol-free boarding house is another crucial part of the service model. People with alcohol-related brain impairment have invariably exhausted the goodwill, patience and endurance of most of their family and friends. As a consequence, the only alternative to transient accommodation options is rooming houses. These have proven to be a mixed bag, some well run and appropriate, but some less so. Paxton is a ten-bed accommodation facility which is run with a view to providing long-standing accommodation for a small group of clients. It had a 99.8 per cent bed occupancy in the 1996/97 financial year. Usually the residents of Paxton are individuals with special needs, including more profound disability or particularly problematic circumstances.

The recreation project

The other initiative we provide is within a special accommodation recreation programme for clients in a series of privately run special accommodation houses (SAHs). Most provide a limited range of recreation options for their residents which begins and ends with turning on the television set. We considered that this was not enough and recruited a group of SAHs who paid a weekly fee for the provision of a recreation worker. This has worked particularly well and has resulted in an ever-increasing list of SAHs who want to participate in the programme.

Case study: Mr C

It is difficult because of the very nature of the disorder and the various medical, psychological and social changes associated with it to form a realistic picture of what individuals who have a diagnosis of WKS go through. The following case provides some small insights into the various effects of the spectrum of the disorder, their implications for the day-to-day activity and the support that ARBIAS gave one man with the problem.

Mr C, aged 57, had been a heavy binge drinker since his 30s. He often drank more than ten units of beer or wine in a session. The episode that brought Mr C to our attention was that he was involved in a motor car accident in which he was hit by a vehicle as a pedestrian. Subsequent to this he claimed that he had no ongoing memory for events. At about this time he left his flat and could not recall the three months prior to his first contact with us. This had resulted in problems with his landlords who were suing him for back rent.

Mr C could only give a sketchy account of his movements over the last few years. He went to Ireland and stayed there for three years. When he came back to Australia he worked at a hotel for about one year and then worked for the council as a groundsman in its gardens for about another year. He could not give any further details after this time, and appeared to have a disruption of recall of events from about 1985 onwards.

Medical investigations revealed that he had a peripheral neuropathy and cerebellar ataxia as well as an associated memory loss. He had no difficulty in performing any of the other tests which are believed to be relatively immune to cerebral insult.

Taken together, the pattern of performance on a range of tests indicates a classic amnesic syndrome of quite severe degree, disruption of pre-existent memories, concreteness of thinking, confabulatory responses and disorientation for time. This pattern is most consistent with WKS. Mr C seemed fairly well preserved, perhaps a little bit more than would be expected at this level of deficit. Nonetheless his cognitive impairment was such that it would have been difficult for him to maintain himself independently at home.

Mr C was referred to the case management service at ARBIAS and was in the first instance put forward to the Guardianship and Administration Board (a government-constituted tribunal responsible for the appointment of guardians and administrators for individuals who are not competent to manage their own financial and personal affairs). The Board considered that Mr C was someone who only required the services of an administrator (an individual who would manage and control his finances), noting that he would need fairly strict supervision regarding his financial, self-care and drinking activities. The issues with the tenancy tribunal were resolved after the nature of the situation was explained to them by the case manager.

Mr C was moved to a more appropriate facility in the form of a special accommodation home where he had contact with a number of younger individuals who had similar problems and needs. He was a keen participant in the recreation activities of the facility, and continues to be to this day.

Conclusion

The medical and psychological problems associated with alcohol intoxication and alcohol withdrawal are due to the ability of alcohol to cause reversible changes in motor and cognitive functioning and to sustain the development of tolerance and physical dependence. Alcohol abuse is associated with several well known neurological diseases including the Wernicke-Korsakoff syndrome (WKS), cerebellar degeneration and peripheral neuropathy (Zubaran, Fernando and Rodnight 1997). More recently, a much wider spectrum of disorders has also been included under the rubric of alcohol-related brain damage (Kopelman 1995; Tuck 1992). Alcoholism, and WKS are not a death sentence. The real work of caring for individuals with ARBI begins after the diagnosis of this problem has been made. The service provision models that we have developed at ARBIAS are one example of how this process might look.

PART THREE

Developing an Individual Understanding

CHAPTER 9

'Dark Head Amongst the Grey'

Experiencing the Worlds
of Younger Persons with Dementia

John Killick

Introduction

There is a sense in which the challenge posed by communicating with those with dementia is not age-related. Many of the ways in which a person with dementia presents him or herself to the potential befriender are the same whether the person is 30, 50 or 70 years old. Among the characteristics I would identify are:

1. short-term memory loss, leading to

2. confusion over the specifics of present place, time and relationships

3. anxiety occasioned by (1) and (2)

4. practical incapacities occasioned by (1), (2) and (3)

5. the use of symbolic language (metaphors, similes, word association) in speech rather than the presentation of logical arguments

6. the eventual breakdown of vocabulary and linguistic structures.

There is a growing literature on communication in this area. Goldsmith (1996) provides an excellent overview of the subject. Of my own texts, the first (Killick 1994) is an explanation of my approach which goes into greater detail than can be attempted here; the second (Killick 1997), whilst expressing a range of emotions and attitudes in the actual words of people with dementia, also provides numerous examples of their use of symbolic language.

Quality of attention

I think by way of introduction it is important to say something about the quality of attention that we give to the person with dementia. Here is what a lady said to me a few weeks ago:

> I want to thank you for listening. You see, YOU ARE WORDS. Words can make or break you. Sometimes people don't listen, they give you words back, and they're all broken, patched up. But will you permit me to say that you have the stillness of silence, that listens and lasts.

She clearly understood what I was doing and revealed the consequences of poor listening. Of course this can be true of anybody in any situation. For a person with dementia, with all the problems that they face, it must be bitterly disappointing to find the effort of attention of the other person lacking, and a distorted meaning attached.

So the quality of attention given is crucial. We cannot expect people with Alzheimer's disease or multi-infarct dementia necessarily to come out and meet us even half way. We who are in full possession of our faculties must do most of the work and provide the patience, consistency and empathy that may be lacking in the other person.

Justification for initiating contact

Of course, some people might say that one has no business intruding on the privacy of such people in the first place. If the world of dementia is a private one we should respect the right of the individual to remain undisturbed in that world. As a care assistant in a nursing home put it to me one day, 'All the people in here' (indicating the lounge area with a sweep of her hand) 'are perfectly happy, and then you come in stirring things up.' This argument might have some force if the people with dementia had chosen the condition in which they find themselves but, since we are speaking of a range of organic brain disorders, that is obviously not the case. The isolation is clearly forced upon them by the nature of the illness, and so it is surely the duty of all of us, who in our different ways have the task of caring for them, to do everything in our power to break down the barriers. And in the initial stages of building a relationship that must involve some degree of 'forcing' our attention upon them.

Once such a move has been made and communication established, it can build at its own pace, as in other relationships, except that one will still have to make steady and prolonged efforts to overcome any problems that may occur. There will, of course, be some individuals who reject or ignore the concentrated attention they are being given, and who may react angrily. I believe that one should persevere to the point where it is clear that there is serious resistance and then withdraw. There may be a personality clash, or this may simply be the wrong time. Persons with dementia often seem to experience wide mood swings, and a rejection one day can be followed by a very different response on another, or even an hour or two later. If you calmly set yourself to get the measure of the situation over a period of time rather than bursting in one moment, and making a once-and-for-all withdrawal the next, you will find that some progress can be made with most people.

In the little book that I wrote for the Dementia Services Development Centre at the University of Stirling (Killick 1994) I spoke of the kind of attention you have to give as 'communicating as if your life depended on it'. This obviously involves a certain amount of exaggeration, but it does make the point that you should not try to make a relationship with a person with dementia unless you are serious about it. There is no point in indulging in trivial chit-chat. It is unlikely to command a response anyway, and it is an insult to the person you are addressing. Somehow you have to empathise and begin to see the world through their eyes. You find the whole of your own personality called upon in the attempt. You are not setting out to impress the other person, only to convince them of your sincerity. And if you are not sincere I believe you will be seen through immediately. I often think that most people with dementia understand far more than we give them credit for. Their problem is more one of giving back responses than of taking in messages in the first place. And because of their language difficulties, which they may well be all too aware of, they are extremely sensitive to atmospheres, to expressions on the face and in the eyes, and to tones of voice.

Silence can be as vital as communication

The lady I quoted at the outset spoke of 'stillness and silence'. In having a conversation with someone with dementia one has to decide what to do about the silences; not yours, those of the other person. Maybe they are occurring because the person has nothing to say. Maybe it is because of the problem of saying anything at all. It is difficult to know. If you feel that it is likely to be the latter (maybe there are stumbling attempts) perhaps you can help by making some suggestions. What you should not do is leap in to fill every gap. If you do that then you become the dominant person in the interaction. The conversation is surely for the benefit of the other person, who lacks your opportunities. How will you ever know what is on *their* mind if you fill the gaps with what is on *your* mind? In order to allow them to set the agenda you must cultivate 'the stillness of silence' – that is, the practice of listening.

I want to offer two more quotations from people I have worked with. They are both commenting on the importance of the quality of communication. The first is highly enthusiastic about the conversation they have just taken part in:

> You're learning a lot, you say, but *I'm* learning so much from *you*: to listen and look so intently and to speak so calmly. Your English is perfect, but mine is no longer perfect: with you I am putting things together. I'm blethering. I don't usually do that, but it's all from beneath the surface. I'm tired, but I don't want to fall asleep because I'm thriving!

The first speaker has concentrated on what is positive about their experience. A second is remembering the failures they have been subjected to:

> I have a problem about kindness. A lot of those who come round here are not interested in being kind to others. Kind is the only thing one can do here. It is all there is that can help. I don't try to be it. You shouldn't have to try to be kind.

Every time I meet someone new who has dementia I remember the first person I quoted: 'YOU ARE WORDS'. It never fails to remind me of the special sense of responsibility that we all bear who work in this area. We are not just there *to do things for them* but *to be with them*. And the way we listen to them, and the way we speak to them, these are the demonstrable signs of our caring.

Case studies

In my preparation for writing this chapter I talked with 18 younger persons with dementia, male and female, in their own homes, in day centres, and in nursing homes. The three I eventually chose to focus on seemed to raise the most issues and to illuminate the characteristics referred to in the introduction. It is axiomatic that all the younger people in the three case studies retain, to a large extent, the ability to reflect upon experience and to formulate their thoughts in coherent sentences. They also make minimal use of symbolic language. In these ways they may well not be seen as typical. However, in the problems which they (and in two cases their carers) elucidate I would suggest that they are indeed representative of the special dilemmas faced by the younger person with dementia. In my concluding section I attempt to draw out some of the issues which must be addressed if the care delivered is to match up to the needs of persons in this age-group. (All names, places and other identifying details in the following studies have been changed to preserve anonymity.)

Case study 1: 'Waging war on patience'

I visited Sam and Brenda in their council flat in the suburb of a large city.

SAM: You must talk as you want to talk with me. I hate secrecy. Brenda says it's a year and a half since I was diagnosed, but I can't remember. Some things I can remember, but it's got to have four legs on it! When I can't remember I get angry. But I know what it's called – Alzheimer's disease.

When I was diagnosed it changed my life completely. They took my licences away because I got in a panic. I'm terrified, and I won't go out in the dark. I keep looking back over my shoulder – I do that even in daylight. I'm diabetic too, but I don't bother with that. And I have cirrhosis. But to tell you the truth I told the doctor I just eat what I want. I don't care because…let's face it …what age am I? …57? …well I've had a good life, so it doesn't matter. But if you can help anyone else…young people especially…I don't consider myself young, not now.

I'm too old for wheels, that's why. What happens with me is that I take notions, and I've an auntie that lives in another part of the city whom I hadn't seen for years. I decided to go and visit her; it must have been some telepathic sense but I got this feeling I had to go. And I set out driving, and that's where the panic started. I couldn't find her, I didn't know where she was. It just took a few minutes. And for years I'd been driving all over Britain. I was even in Aden. It was a brand-new lorry and it seized up. It was only the Commandos that sorted me out…Sandra, the mental health officer, came in regularly. And she asked me to go to a resource centre for four weeks. I said I'd go, but that I'd come back here because nobody's going to push me about. They were all old people, they were really old, I'm telling you. Actually two of them died who were round the corner. After four weeks I said 'That'll do – it's not for me'. I was still driving at that time…

What happened was this, and I'm going to tell the truth. It was my son that made me panic. He was the one that tipped me over the edge. They stopped me anyway, and that hurts, because there must be 90 million people still doing it. I can assure you that I've got a cousin, and he's got Alzheimer's, and he sneaks off to the pub, and then he's driving. He's been driving lorries for years. And there's others whose names I could give you too. I feel angry about this!

BRENDA: Well it was really that when you went on an anti-depressant you couldn't drive because it ruins your concentration.

SAM: It was a big blow to me because it was my life. And it wasn't just one licence, it was three that was taken off me – my car licence, my HGV licence, and my PSV licence – I lost them all at one go.

I could do everything once; now I can do nothing. Not since the panicking. I tell you, I was in the desert once, with Arabs all around me, and I lay there. There was a gun but no bullets. I was not in fear then, nothing...I tell you, I did walk the dog, but not any more. I've not been over the door for two weeks come Saturday. I just don't want to do it. If I go anywhere I go with her [indicating Brenda].

BRENDA: And we have more arguments when we're out than we do when we're here!

SAM: Listen, I loved it out, I loved it down the markets. But without the car you've got to walk for miles. I knew what to do, it was to get a bus and change. And the reason I remembered it was Uncle Joe was staying here, and we went there. Now I watch every move. I keep looking to see where I'm going. I follow the same routes...

BRENDA: Tell about the day when we went on the bus to the markets.

SAM: Oh I'm telling you, that was a laugh – I'm not kidding you! It took hours! That wasn't my fault, that was the bus! It goes round every scheme there is!

BRENDA: You won't get off any stop before the end because that's what you've paid for! And then we had to walk miles. By the time we was getting to the markets they was shutting!

SAM: I still went!

BRENDA: We finally get in, and they was packing all their stuff up! What a carry on! We laughed after it but at the time it was frustrating. All we had got was something to eat because I was worried about the diabetes. You know, one of the things with Alzheimer's is everything's got to be done like yesterday. Before he would have took his time doing things, but now if he's too long, like going on a journey, he'll not go back there. He's much more impatient.

He doesn't go in the betting shop because he's fallen out with the people so I'm putting the line on and he's standing outside. If I say maybe we should go up the street and here and there, he won't want to go. If I suggest it, it's no go. He's got to be there on the spot or not at all. It's a kind of waging war on patience. That's the way I'm seeing it.

SAM: I worked as a lorry driver, and I loved this firm. My boss was the best man you could ever work for. And I tell you, I miss it, that life, and I miss him! I was like a gypsy – on my own, I'd sleep in the cab, I had my own television and everything in it, I used to smoke 60 Bensons a day – yes, I really miss that, and I miss the man!

I was away so much, but now I'm here all the time. But Brenda still rules! I do a lot here – I clean up and everything. And I shift the house about. I shifted that cabinet myself.

BRENDA: One day I went out and when I came back the stairs were painted black! He takes a notion to paint, and then everything gets done. But he misses parts and just leaves them, he doesn't go back to them again. He painted before, but just things like the window sills.

There have been other big changes for me. The night I've to go to the bingo he falls out with me that day. He gets into a bad mood because I go out. I'm supposed to look after him 24 hours a day!

SAM: Well it's a very lonely life.

BRENDA: But you've made it lonely yourself, because you've cut yourself off from everybody! You used to spend a few hours down the betting shop – it gave you an interest. You used to leave here about one o'clock and come back at five.

SAM: I stopped going because he was fiddling me. I said 'Peter, if I have one halfpenny short in my money (I couldn't count it myself any longer) I'll be on the phone to head office, it isn't right'. I hate anything like that. But I don't want to use any other betting shop. So I send Brenda. I couldn't go anywhere else. I keep looking round – I wouldn't feel safe.

It's very lonely, I'm telling you. We have a large family, but we don't talk about it. I don't want the grandchildren to know, not until it gets really bad, then I'd rather get put away somewhere. I was actually going to walk away last week. I don't know what it was about. I was going to walk away from the loneliest life in the world. Although you're here, you can't get into company. You get this thing in your head and it switches off, and you're left nowhere. It's just like switching the light out, and it's terrible.

I was the most happy-go-lucky fellow. I used to go down to the club and the pub and drink whisky. Now I don't want to go out. And I don't want anyone coming in here. I weigh people up. I'm watching them. In my position, the way that I feel, I don't have trust. And I was never like that.

Case study 2: 'Lots of money but little intimacy'

I had visited this nursing home once before and had experienced the beginnings of a relationship with Mary, who had been admitted only a few days previously. On that occasion she was in a very distressed state, always on the move, and showing a marked reluctance to speak with staff or other residents. She held my hand, however, and allowed me to walk with her. She spoke with me, but seemed only to be able to manage isolated sentences. I was returning to the home a fortnight later, at the request of the matron, specifically to try to build on the rapport already established, in an attempt to help Mary to become reconciled to her new surroundings. My journal takes up the tale…

Wednesday. I arrive at about 7.00 p.m., let myself in and come onto the unit. Almost the first person I see is Mary. She passes the end of the corridor walking purposefully, then doubles back, having caught a glimpse of me. She comes towards me smiling, holding her hands out. I take them and we kiss. Immediately we start walking. She goes up to the first resident that we see and says 'This is the gentleman. He's come back.' We continue on our walk.

I talk about where I have been since I last saw her, mentioning my wife and children, different pieces of work completed. She says nothing, but occasionally smiles in a private sort of way. I ask her what has been happening to her. 'Nothing really.' Has she received my postcards? 'I don't think so.' She remembers which is my room (I stay on the unit when visiting). A care assistant brings the key. Mary enters before me, turning the lights on, moving things about. She takes things from me as I unpack, hanging them and putting them in drawers. She takes her own coat off and hangs it behind the door. Suddenly she hears another resident's voice in the corridor. 'Your friend, he needs you.' She takes my hand and guides it into the other resident's. He says 'I'm having an operation tomorrow to improve my eyes'. 'Oh, I'm sorry' – Mary smiles sympathetically. She leads me back into my room, and takes the bangles off her wrist, placing them on the dressing table. All the agitation seems, at least temporarily, to have left her. 'I'm hungry,' I say. 'I'd better go and find some tea. Are you coming with me?' 'No, I've had mine.' She accompanies me along the corridor. When I turn left towards the kitchens she marches straight forward, face set grim with determination.

In the staff room I find a postcard addressed to her. I bring it back with me. She reads out, '"I was glad to speak to you on the phone on Sunday".' 'Who is it from?' 'Alice and Arthur. My friends.' She returns with me to my room, and I prop the door open. Whilst I eat Mary slips her shoes off and climbs on the bed. She lies on her side with her eyes wide open; she seems calm and relaxed. 'That's my bed, you know,' I say. 'Yes.' 'What am I supposed to do?' She grins and closes her eyes. 'Find another one.' When she starts to snore two care assistants arrive and help her back to her own room and put her to bed.

Thursday. I have already had my breakfast when she appears, kisses me, and lets me lead her to the dining room. Afterwards we begin some serious walking. The matron has opened fire doors on two sides of the building so that Mary can go in and out freely, but this is insufficient for her. With characteristic foolhardiness I suggest taking Mary out for a walk.

The matron agrees. When we get to the bottom of the drive Mary breaks into a run, still holding my hand. 'Where are we going?'

'Home.' 'Where is home?' 'Farleigh.' At a road junction we stop. I'm glad because I'm quite out of breath. 'Which way?' I ask. It is clear that neither of us knows. Mary drops my hand and for a moment I'm afraid she is going to run away. To my astonishment she sets off back to the nursing home, arriving before me.

We eat lunch together. She only gets up six times during the meal; usually it is at least twice that number. She eats very discreetly compared with the other residents (all at least twenty years older than her). The only other sign of confusion is when she piles table mats and utensils on top of each other.

In the evening Mary's friend Grace arrives to see her, but she refuses to talk to her unless I am present. Grace indicates that she wishes to speak to me alone, and waits until Mary has gone to bed. 'She seems to have a closer relationship with you than anyone,' she says 'so I want to tell you everything I know about her, which may help to explain why she is so unhappy.'

She tells me that Mary, who is now 56 years old, is the only child of very correct parents who lived in a large mansion. She received an expensive private education. Her father was a professional man; he died seventeen years ago, and her mother was only to survive him by ten years. Before he died her father asked a doctor, Dr W, for whom Mary worked as private secretary, to look after her. There are no relatives, apart from two cousins, who live in Scotland. Work for Mary has been the centre of her life, her social contacts have been extremely limited: she has never been 'permitted' a boy-friend. After her mother's death she lived on in the big house alone. Her behaviour became erratic: sometimes she would arrive very late for work, or not turn up at all. Once she arrived several hours early for a doctor's appointment. It was after Dr W's retirement that things deteriorated further. She didn't seek other employment and became 'a complete loner'. Friends felt that she 'blanked herself off' and at times behaved in a 'paranoid' fashion. She accused the neighbours of prying – trying to watch her when she took baths, for instance; she would phone Grace up to ten times a day with complaints. Eventually the police were involved.

Dr W's wife persuaded Mary to invite her relatives from Scotland to stay because she wanted their opinion about her condition. They found the house in a very disorganised state, and while they were there Mary collapsed with 'a fit' and was admitted to hospital. She was given a magnetic resonance imaging (MRI) and computerised tomography (CT) scan and also an electroencephalography (EEG) which showed an abnormality. The only residential accommodation available was this nursing home, and so she was admitted. When the house was cleared a journal was found detailing numerous migraines and many of the symptoms of dementia.

Grace says that she is probably Mary's best friend, but doesn't feel that she has ever really got close to her. She sums up Mary's life in the following words 'lots of money but little intimacy'. She has always been used to freedom and isolation so her reaction to the curtailment of her liberty was predictable. If she had any close relatives living this would have provided a more positive caring alternative, but lacking that option the best hope must lie in building other relationships. Not easy when her co-residents are much older than her, though in her case she has always been used to the company of older people.

Friday. I am leaving this morning. Mary appears reconciled to it. Over breakfast we talk about when I will make my next visit; I promise that it will be no more than a week or two away. I arrange a schedule of postcards, phone calls and tapes, punctuated by visits, which will continue (I tell myself) until she has formed relationships with residents and staff and hopefully become more integrated into the life of the home.

Case study 3: 'Realising I'm only here once, and making the most of it'

I visited Phil and Sandra in their town centre flat.

JOHN: Are you able to get around now by yourself?

PHIL: No.

JOHN: Why is that? How does it affect you?

PHIL: I'm all right going, but something happens coming back. I don't have the wherewithal to come back.

JOHN: So does the concentration go at some point? You can't remember the way?

PHIL: Yes.

JOHN: And how do you feel when that happens?

PHIL: Panicky. Sometimes when we go shopping I'm sat on a seat, and maybe she takes a long time. Panic. Where is she? Has she gone home without me? It's not rational. It's a feeling, and it comes from yourself. Years ago I wouldn't have bothered. I'd have gone there by myself in any case.

JOHN: So you don't put yourself in those situations if you can help it?

PHIL: No.

JOHN: So, Sandra, that means that wherever Phil wants to go you've got to go too?

SANDRA: Yes.

JOHN: And wherever you want to go...

SANDRA: I've got to take him with me. I wouldn't even leave him in the house because he's a danger to himself. I mean, if he's forgotten where I've gone... The furthest I've gone is that I've jumped in the car to go to the garage for cigarettes at night, ten minutes at the most. Or maybe to take my mother home.

PHIL: Even then, I'd begin worrying... Where's she gone?

SANDRA: I can't leave him because I would worry that he would come out looking for me. But not only that: he doesn't know how to operate the video. He can switch on the telly, that's all.

JOHN: But, Phil, you give the impression of being so capable.

PHIL: But I'm not. I'm OK sitting here, but...

JOHN: I saw you in the day centre and I got the impression that you were really good at coping.

PHIL: That's when I'm with people. But I can't be on my own before I begin to get panicky.

SANDRA: I think this is part of a general problem with younger sufferers. They look perfectly normal. They sound perfectly normal. To see Phil at the pool table you would never know that there's anything wrong with him. But ask him what he had for his lunch and he couldn't tell you.

John: Why is it, Phil, that you can remember how to play pool but not how to switch on the video?

SANDRA: That's easily explained. Pool, his trade, various things that he's done – these are from his younger days, and he can remember them...

PHIL: But video, that's all new to me, and I can't get the hang of it.

SANDRA: Take money. Five pence, for example.

PHIL: It's all the decimalisation. I can only remember pennies.

SANDRA: But he can recognise pound coins. I can't give him notes, because of old they went in your back pocket. Well he'll put them in there, and draw them out with his comb and lose them.

JOHN: Can I ask you, Phil, how long have you had dementia?

PHIL: Haven't a clue. [*Laughs*]

SANDRA: It'll be about six and a half years ago when he was actually diagnosed. Phil has Korsakoff's...

PHIL: And he should bloody well have kept it! [*All laugh*]

SANDRA: There's a question mark over multi-infarct. It first came to light with a stroke over the brain. They took him into hospital without realising, and immediately blamed it on the alcohol. They kept him in for nearly two weeks and then were going to send him home. I said 'I'm sorry, but there's something very far wrong here'. Although he sounded plausible enough he was talking a whole load of piddle.

PHIL: I could flannel my way out of anything.

SANDRA: They transferred him to the psychiatric unit, and a psychiatrist did the further diagnosis. Since then he's had a couple more strokes. All this has affected his ability to get around. Phil himself recognises that people will accept physical disability more readily than mental.

JOHN: Phil, how do you feel about the way people accept you?

PHIL: Most of the people I'm in contact with accept me. I'm either with people who understand, or if I'm not and someone asks me a question I can't answer I say 'Ask the wife'.

SANDRA: That's not what you say at all.

Phil: What do I say then?

SANDRA: You say 'Ask the boss'! [*All laugh*]

PHIL: I push it away from me. I rely on someone else's answer.

SANDRA: I think too, though, that as the illness progresses this can bring its own difficulties. There is now a lack of inhibitions, so very often what Phil says is the first thing that comes into his head, and sometimes it's not the right thing to say. It can put you in quite embarrassing positions.

JOHN: Do you think there are any plusses in losing inhibitions? We are most of us too inhibited, aren't we?

SANDRA: In some ways. I'll give you an example. There's a baker's shop in the town, and behind it there's a tea room. We were there on this day and they've had problems with school kids coming in to use the toilets, so they've taken the keys and put them behind the till. You leave a pound deposit to get a key. And this man of mine stands up in the middle of the tea-room and announces to the entire population therein 'This is the dearest place in town for a pee'! [*All laugh*]

PHIL: There's another point here, though. I can lay my pound down for a key but I might forget to take it back to them. The key would be lost to them, and I would have lost my pound!

SANDRA: But this is where you meet difficulties as well. Isn't it funny how in an elderly person who comes away with something which can either be nasty or rude people are very indulgent and will say 'Oh, never mind'. But for Phil to do that is highly unacceptable. The line is drawn in a different place. You might say that the accommodations for dementia sufferers are geared up for elderly people. Phil has quite a childlike sense of humour, and that for me is one of his qualities – it's lovely. So for Phil in the respite situation we've got, the other patients think he's one of the staff. He looks younger, he has a quick wit, and he doesn't seem to fit with the rest of the group.

PHIL: What we need – those of us in my situation – is opportunities for recreation. I'll do anything where I can be with other folk. I need to feel accepted, and there has to be something to show for it. See that stool there? – I made it in the day centre. They took me out into the town and I bought the stuff in a craft shop. Then they advised me how to go on with it.

SANDRA: I held out for a long time over sending Phil to respite, but then I realised I was being silly. If I went down with anything he'd have to go anyway. But I still have misgivings. His main complaint when I bring him home is 'Nobody talks to you'.

PHIL: Not a word. You have no conversation with the other patients because they don't come to you and you don't go to them. The staff are all right, but they're only there to look after you, they don't have time to sit and talk. Conversation is part of your life, and if it's not there you miss it. But the way it is, you feel as if they've sat you there and left you there for good.

SANDRA: This is an important point. When elderly people are diagnosed they have probably been retired for a number of years, and they have got into a way of life which is more suited, perhaps, to accepting this sitting back and doing very little. But when a younger person is diagnosed you are very often taking them out of a workplace situation and a social life and you are handing them nothing in return.

JOHN: Do you miss work, Phil?

PHIL: Oh yes. I was a compositor, setting up type. I took an apprenticeship. But latterly that trade packed up, and I've done a variety of things: taxi driver, bus conductor...

JOHN: Can I ask how old you are?

PHIL: Sixty-two nearly. Well 31 really – my twin-brother has the other 31! [*All laugh*] He's still working.

SANDRA: But he's a painter and decorator and he's had very little work over the past year. Phil has the life of Riley compared with him!

JOHN: I want to ask you, Sandra, if having Phil at home with you all the time has brought good times as well as bad?

SANDRA: Oh yes. But you have to take this individually. I mean, there are some people with the illness where the personality change is for the worse. In Phil's case, being an alcoholic brought out the worst in him. I'm now seeing the man I first met as a teenager...

PHIL: Rejuvenation!

Sandra: ...so that's a bonus.

JOHN: He seems such a nice guy.

SANDRA: He was. He is. But alcohol changed all that. He became a Mr Nasty guy.

JOHN: Can you remember what it was like when you were drinking heavily?

PHIL: No. You just go on to the next drink. You think you're great.

SANDRA: In actual fact, when Phil was diagnosed he and I had been separated for six years. I was living in a different town. The one thing that kept us going was that first and foremost we are very good friends. I couldn't live with him, I had to let go, but then this happened. He was in the hospital for six months, and when they diagnosed Korsakoff's we were told he would be put in an institution because there was no way he could carry on with his life by himself. From that day forward he never had another drink. Then after his heart attack he hasn't smoked either. But during the alcoholic years I suffered the kind of treatment that I now see other people suffering at the hands of people with the illness. I had one wife say to me 'You are so lucky that Phil has gone the way he's gone. My husband's personality has changed so that he abuses me and uses foul language and tries to hit me.' And I said 'Yes, but I've been there.'

JOHN: Surely, physically you live more closely than you've ever done? Would it be true to say that in other ways you are closer too?

SANDRA: Well, Phil is totally dependent upon me. But at the same time I'm dependent upon him for a lot of things – just making me laugh, keeping me right, company. Of course he can be very stubborn and dig his heels in, which is quite difficult, and he doesn't trust, but apart from that, he doesn't have mood changes.

PHIL: I've seen other folk getting conned. I've seen things end in fisticuffs. So I don't trust them. Putting your trust in strangers, that's what I used to do. Now I've really got to get to know people before I can begin to trust them. The only person I trust all the time is Sandra.

SANDRA: And there's a sense in which he can only trust me when he can see me. When I'm in the supermarket he'll sit in the tea shop, but I have to make sure that I come into his view as often as I come down the aisle, otherwise he gets frightened.

JOHN: Obviously the dementia is progressive. How slow or fast is it in Phil's case?

SANDRA: Korsakoff's itself seems slow, they can last for ever. But with the multi-infarct you are getting these small impulses all the time and you hardly know they're happening. The only clue you have to it is that, say it has happened during the night, well in the morning the speech is slurred, or his mouth is twisted, and these right themselves. But I feel that each time something more is lost. The doctors keep telling me that it doesn't necessarily do any harm, but I have to disagree. Each time, though it comes back, it doesn't quite come back.

PHIL: Yes, memory – another little bit of memory lost. But I've got quality of life. I'm realising I'm only here once, and making the most of it!

SANDRA: The psychiatrist said, when I was bringing Phil home six years ago, that it can't be done, that what I've done can't be done.

JOHN: How have you achieved it?

SANDRA: Well, I listen to the other carers, and I think maybe I have a better deal because I chose to go into this situation, whereas it has been flung upon them and there's quite a bit of resentment. But, accepting that, then I think it's the realisation that you have to motivate all the time. So I suppose I'd say it's the one-to-one.

JOHN: I think what you've proved is that the one-to-one is so positive, it's a force to be reckoned with.

SANDRA: Absolutely.

PHIL: Yes, *she's* a force to be reckoned with! [*All laugh*]

Conclusion

There is no doubt in my mind, after spending time in a concentrated attempt to 'enter the world' of the younger person with dementia, that special emphasis needs to be put on aspects of communicating with this age group.

First of all, many younger persons do appear to have a greater awareness of their condition than is found amongst older people. Both Sam and Phil know what they are suffering from and can enumerate its effects upon their lives. The same might well be true of Mary if her level of anxiety was not so extreme.

Sam speaks of 'the loneliest life in the world' but most of the time his terrors are held at bay by the security offered by Brenda, and by a conscious attempt to avoid putting himself in situations where his inadequacies will be tested.

Phil adopts similar strategies; he appears to lean more heavily on his wife and take strength from the constant support Sandra offers, but also to have reserves of his own, through humour and subterfuge, so that he is able to speak positively of his 'quality of life'.

So there is a remarkable degree of self-awareness being exercised in two out of three of these individuals, though this may be due to earlier diagnosis in younger people. Sam and Phil both comment about the hurts caused to their sensibilities by having to mix with older people for social activities/respite.

Awareness provides the possibility of greater understanding, and therefore of surviving more effectively. It can lead to depression (and Sam seems close to that) because of the greater potentiality for distress to be felt. All three experience terror at one time or another. Sam and Phil both use the same word for it: 'panic'. Mary rushing to find an exit is in an almost constant state of panic, and at the end of each day she virtually collapses from emotional and physical exhaustion. People can, however, be helped to devise strategies for coping. In the case of the two men their marriages act as life belts which help to save them from the sea of confusion surrounding them. Mary has no such rescue service available, hence the importance of building up relationships. This seems to be happening within the home.

Some people who cannot cope with the reality of their situation appear to deny their problem. Over half of those I spoke to in depth appeared to show signs of this characteristic. Since it is unrepresented in the three illustrations I have provided, here is part of a conversation I had with Alan in a day centre.

JOHN: How old are you?

ALAN: My age is…that is a…damned if I can think of…well, less than 60…I can't…born here, in this town… My father was…can't remember. He was a lorry-driver once…that's it… that's just one of those things… that's stuck in my mind.

JOHN: Do you have problems with remembering?

ALAN: Well it's hard to say…hard to say about remembering…it was…a long time ago… Mum and dad died… I got married… I have a son…and grandsons…to ensure the line… I prefer…to have ensurance of young blood.

JOHN: What is this place?

ALAN: It's a place…to give purpose to people, I suppose… They're…not bad here… I don't know if I'd come more often… that's if I could.

JOHN: You don't work now, do you?

ALAN: I don't work now, no. I'm not…retired…but I wouldn't want it, want my job back.

JOHN: Can you remember your age now?

ALAN: No. I feel as young as my dogs… Alsatians, aye.

This is fairly typical of a number of the conversations which took place. It is hard to put one's finger on it but I have the distinct impression from such exchanges that the memory problems demonstrated are not just by-products of the disease, but serve a more strategic function of keeping consideration of the dementia at arm's length. In other words, they ward off the questioner but they also provide an excuse for the individual so that he/she is shielded from the full realisation of what is happening to them. This is a matter of extreme delicacy, and just as one would not dream of prodding a physical wound, I think one should not attempt to disturb the precarious equilibrium, although supportive relationships may still be formed.

Younger people with dementia are often much closer in age to the central concerns of their lives than older people, so it is no surprise to find that Sam and Phil are still very involved in family events and relationships. They also experience a proximity to their working roles, and both voice a keen sense of loss in this area. In Sam this deprivation centres upon the withdrawal of his driving licences.

But perhaps the most striking characteristic which emerges from all three illustrations is the emphasis on trust. The word is used by both men, and it is clear that the onset of dementia has been accompanied by serious losses in this area. They are hanging on tenaciously to what in either case they believe is the one relationship which has not failed them, but the ever-present fear of loss of control over their environment continues to place even that under suspicion. In Mary we see the first tentative attempts to recapture the benefits of a trusting relationship.

In a recent paper on a psychotherapeutic approach to listening to the stories that people with dementia tell, Sutton and Cheston (1997, p.162) make the following sensitive observations:

> We are listening to people talking about a pain that may well one day be our own or that of our husbands, wives, fathers and mothers. We cannot make this future 'better' in the sense of taking this pain away; we can only try and listen and to help the person feel that they have been heard. This is as hard as it is necessary.

As I emerge from a period of intense listening to the words of younger people with dementia, people not far removed from myself in age, I feel I have even greater cause to reflect upon the difficulty (intense pain) and the necessity (urgency) of the process.

CHAPTER 10

Negotiating Caregiving and Employment

Diane Seddon

Introduction

Studies on the relationship between employment and caregiving, as experienced by informal carers, remains sparse. This chapter is based on a recent qualitative study of carers of younger people with dementia. It intends to sensitise readers to the dynamics involved in negotiating the demands of caregiving and employment and to the carers' expertise in managing the broad range of activities. Drawing upon case material provided from their accounts, various management strategies are discerned and specific difficulties identified. An appraisal of the impact, relevance and effectiveness of supportive interventions then follows. Drawing upon carers' expert knowledge, the chapter provides useful pointers for policy and practice, identifies shortfalls in provision, prioritises areas for improvement and reinforces the need to devise age-sensitive interventions. It begins by presenting an overview of the literature, identifying the key concepts and theoretical models which gave direction to the study.

Informal caregiving: A growing concern

In recent years there has been a burgeoning of studies relating to the provision of informal care and the position of the informal carer. Focusing primarily upon familial support of dependent population groups, for instance, parents looking after their disabled children (Beresford 1994), spouses caring for their physically disabled partner (Parker 1993) and daughters caring for their elderly mothers (Lewis and Meredith 1988), studies have confirmed that caregiving can have detrimental consequences in a

number of areas of functioning. The most pervasive effects have been identified in relation to the carers' emotional well being, their physical health and
their social and family life. Set against this, there is growing evidence that the
stresses and strains of caregiving are often juxtaposed with a sense of purpose, meaning and identity (Nolan, Grant and Keady 1996).

Partly in response to research findings, the support needs of carers and the
appropriateness of various interventions have been subject to debate (Twigg
and Atkin 1994). Occupying an uncertain and ambiguous position, carers
are often not recognised as legitimate service recipients. Services are generally directed towards meeting the needs of dependants, are frequently
delivered in irrational and discriminatory ways and remain crisis oriented.

Recent thinking on interventions with carers has been strongly influenced by the transactional model of stress and coping which stems from the
work of Lazarus (1966). Underpinning the model is the concept of subjective appraisal, the cognitive process whereby an individual assesses whether a
demand threatens their well being and appraises their resources for meeting
the demand. Within this model, the presence of an individual with dementia
is not viewed as an inevitable burden. Rather, it acts as a potential stressor
which impacts upon the well being of the carer and is mediated by his or her
coping strategies. Having proved powerful in explaining variations of stress
amongst carers and exploring individual circumstances, the transactional
model holds considerable potential for devising interventions which are tailored to carers' specific requirements.

A substantial body of literature on the instrumental aspects of caring, for
instance the daily routines of carers, has accumulated and the UK is now
entering a second phase of caregiving research (Phillips 1995). The
long-term consequences of assuming the caring role are beginning to be
addressed, as are the difficulties faced by particular groups of carers. In recent
years the needs of people with early onset dementia and their carers have
become more apparent (Cox and McLennan 1994). However, only isolated
studies have addressed the personal, service and practice issues involved in
caring for this group. This limited attention may be attributed to two factors;
the lack of nationally representative epidemiological data and the absence of
a theoretical framework identifying the particular needs of those who
acquire dementia in middle age (Keady and Nolan 1994). Consequently,
there is little evidence of a coordinated approach to this group's needs,
younger people with dementia and their carers remaining 'orphaned in
no-man's land' (Williams 1995, p.699).

Due to the non-normative timing of their experience, carers of younger people with dementia face different life conditions than their elderly counterparts. They may have young children or adolescents living at home (Quinn 1996) and are more likely to be in employment (Alzheimer's Disease Society 1995) and to have considerable financial commitments, such as a mortgage. It is their employment commitments and the complex organizational issues involved in their caregiving role which comprise the focus of this chapter.

Caregiving and employment

Carers in employment

Employment status is an important sociodemographic variable associated with the provision of informal care, having significant implications for the future supply of carers, the quality of care provided and the carer's preference for institutionalisation. Of the six million informal carers in the UK, three million are carer-workers. These carers are known to spend an equivalent number of hours providing care as their non-employed counterparts. A consideration of such factors as increased life expectancy, the rising median age of the labour force and the increase in female labour market participation would suggest that the number of employed carers is set to increase.

From a consideration of the available research it is clear that caring responsibilities can impact upon employment in a variety of ways and that carers often fail to realise their full potential in the labour market (Evandrou 1995). The restriction upon the number of hours they are able to devote to employment coupled with geographical immobility, difficulties in pursuing formal training and sensitivity to the needs of the dependant limit the types of employment carers are able to undertake and impede career development during the critical years. Many are forced to make alterations to their working lives, including transferring from full-time to part-time employment, resigning and 'opting' for early retirement.

The effects of caregiving upon employment are not distributed equally between men and women, with men reporting fewer consequences in terms of job and career effects (Martin Matthews and Campbell 1995). Similarly, carers assisting dependants between the ages of 18 and 64 years are thought to experience higher levels of strain than those caring for an elderly parent (Neal et al. 1993). To date, comparatively little attention has been devoted to this group, previous studies having relied primarily upon data from caregivers of older people.

Combining employment and care

Whilst most carers are able to negotiate their dual roles, the pressures involved in managing the spillover are immense and the costs, in terms of stress and absenteeism, are high. Those caring for a cognitively impaired person are thought to experience particularly high levels of stress and work interference (Scharlach 1989).

At an individual level, the process of negotiation is influenced by a number of factors, ranging from societal norms and values, to the structure and dynamics of the family, the availability of support and the attitude of employers. Carers in different occupations have differing opportunities available to them for adjusting their caregiving and work demands, the range of options reflecting seniority and autonomy as well as formal workplace policies.

Leaving employment

Caring is itself a job and one which may prove so onerous that carers are left with little option other than to withdraw from employment. Evidence indicates that an increasing number are confronted with this dilemma.

The consequences of leaving employment are serious in both the short term and the long term, resulting in what McLaughlin and Ritchie (1994, p.241) refers to as the 'legacies of caring'. In the present economic climate the prospects of re-entering the labour market are poor and what may have been perceived as a temporary break in employment may eventually turn out to be permanent retirement. The impact varies and is dependent upon the carer's stage in the lifecycle. Ex-carers who do return may face lower rates of pay due to a loss of seniority and a lack of up-to-date work experience. Most difficult to quantify are the costs in relation to the carer's social and emotional well being. Employment often serves as a necessary counterbalance to caregiving, providing carers with an emotional outlet and a structured opportunity to meet others. Those who leave often experience a sense of isolation, increased levels of stress and depression and a loss of self-esteem.

Employment policies

Recently, there have been calls for employers to introduce greater flexibility into work practices, for example flexitime and job sharing. Despite these calls, research into 'carer-friendly' employment practices reveals that work patterns remain inflexible and that employer attitudes are characterised by 'structural thoughtlessness' (Naegele and Reichert 1995, p.85). This is surprising as, given the opportunity, carers may bring valuable attributes to the workplace, for example interpersonal and managerial skills.

Changes in employment policies alone are insufficient to protect carers' employment. Comprehensive and flexible support services are also required. At present, balancing employment and caregiving is not supported by policy initiatives or service provision, carer employment issues having been virtually ignored in national policy and practice guidance (DoH 1989; Social Services Inspectorate 1991a) and in debates concerning the promotion of equal opportunities. In terms of services, provision discriminates against carers in paid employment.

Individual experiences of caregiving

Sixteen case studies were conducted in the county of Gwynedd, North Wales. Evidence gathered for the case studies was derived from a series of semi-structured interviews in which carers were accorded considerable freedom to report their experiences at length and in their own words. Subject to written consent, interviews were tape recorded and transcribed. An in-depth analysis of the data was subsequently undertaken.

The choice of cases was made on conceptual rather than representative grounds, each being selected from the caseload of a consultant psychiatrist. Caring for a relative with a diagnosis of Alzheimer's disease, the subjects recruited were either spouses or adult children who were co-resident or providing care to the relative in their own home. The sample included four carers of younger people with dementia. It is the lived experiences of this small sub-group, introduced below, which will comprise the focus of the chapter.

All names have been changed to preserve anonymity.

Mrs Brown

Mrs Brown is 46 years old and cares for her husband, aged 54. Married for 28 years, they have a daughter and three grandchildren. A sprightly lady with a strong sense of duty, Mrs Brown has looked after her husband for three years. She resigned from full-time employment 12 months after the diagnosis.

Described by his wife as 'moderately demented', Mr Brown lacks self-care skills and has continence problems. He experiences difficulties in conversing, is extremely irascible and no longer recognises his wife.

Apart from three days at the day centre and a weekly visit from the district nurse, Mrs Brown receives a minimum of service provision. This is despite her own deteriorating health.

Mrs Crosby

At 19 years of age Mrs Crosby is the youngest carer in the study, caring for her 41-year-old mother. Married with a young son, she provides constant care to her doubly incontinent, non-ambulatory and partially blind mother who has had Alzheimer's disease for three years. Overwhelmed by the responsibility and worried as to the long-term effects on her son, Mrs Crosby left full-time employment several weeks prior to the first interview. She receives regular provision of formal support which includes day care and home help.

Mr Davies

Mr Davies is 57 years old and cares for his wife, aged 65. Married for 34 years, they have two sons, the youngest of whom lives at home. Mrs Davies had Alzheimer's disease for six years and is crippled with rheumatoid arthritis. She requires complete assistance with activities of daily living. A devoted husband, Mr Davies resigned from his job in desk-top publishing 18 months prior to the first interview.

In terms of support, Mrs Davies attends day care on Mondays, a district nurse visits twice weekly and a home help visits every other day. At the time of the second interview she lived in permanent care. Fatigued and experiencing great difficulty in coming to terms with the sequence of events, Mr Davies is actively seeking employment.

Mrs Smith

Mrs Smith is 54 years old and looks after her husband, aged 59. Married for 34 years, they have three children. Mr Smith was diagnosed as having Alzheimer's disease following a series of incidents involving the police. Previously, his paranoid and aggressive behaviour, which had spanned a period of four years, had been attributed to depression.

Diagnosed as having severe dementia, Mr Smith requires complete assistance with activities of daily living. Restless and disoriented, he is prone to catastrophic reactions. Initially, he attended day care twice weekly. This was increased to four days shortly after Mrs Smith left work. A home help visits three days a week and a Crossroads care attendant visits on two afternoons.

By the time of the second interview Mr Smith lived in permanent care and was not expected to live long. Mesmerised by her predicament, Mrs Smith had returned to part-time employment.

The intention of these brief portraits is to enable readers to secure subsequent discussions to a fixed point of reference and relate the themes identified to 'real-life' situations.

The following themes and concepts are suggested as a tentative framework with which to understand more fully some of the key issues. Formulated and refined on the basis of evidence from the wider sample of 16 case studies, the qualitative perspective of younger onset carers is captured through narrative descriptions and attention is paid to the particular difficulties they face.

Adopting a proactive stance

Engaging in problem focused coping (Lazarus and Folkman 1984), carers devise schedules within which they strive to negotiate their caring and employment responsibilities. Designed to bring a semblance of orderliness and organisation into daily life, they provide the framework within which carers cope. An integral part of their daily routine, there is unanimous agreement that without a schedule of some description employment would not be feasible.

> You have to have a schedule, that's paramount me dear and you have 'ta be able to, erm, how can I put it, prioritise things within that schedule. If you didn't work things out like that you'd never cope... You never knew how she was goin' to be an' so you didn't work it out to the letter, er, you'd sort'a do somethin' up like, some sort of schedule and try to keep to it as close you could. I did a few rough ones on paper first... They'd get thrown out a bit but nothin' you couldn't compensate for. (Mr Davies)

Subject to continuous appraisal, schedules are refined to accommodate the progression of the dependants' condition and the dynamic circumstances under which carers operate.

Charting schedule development

Recognising the importance of organisation and planning, two carers, Mrs Brown and Mrs Smith, appraised the resources at their disposal and formulated schedules at an early stage. In contrast, Mrs Crosby and Mr Davies adopted a piecemeal approach, their schedules having evolved after they had been in danger of becoming overwhelmed by their circumstances. Previous attempts at negotiating responsibilities were blighted by disorganisation and fragmentation, both having faced a barrage of unpunctuated demands which they were able to make little sense of.

Schedule components

Negotiating the demands of caregiving and employment involves a broad spectrum of activities, ranging from the necessities of existence to optional recreational activities. Essentially, schedules comprise five constituent parts including time allotted to:

- dependant care
- employment
- household(s) maintenance
- personal needs
- other family members.

At the necessity end of the spectrum, carers prioritise dependant care and employment. Concessions are made with respect to the maintenance of the home. The fourth and fifth components are judged the most expendable, carers compromising the time reserved for attending to personal needs, for example, pursuing outside interests, and for other family members. But how do carers set about managing their schedules on a daily basis?

Schedule management

The term 'management strategy' is used to describe what carers do on a practical level during the course of conducting their daily lives. A number of strategies are discerned and considered under three broad headings:

- the organisation of time
- the use of time
- frameworks of support.

Largely taken for granted and adopted almost unconsciously, strategies are rarely used on an individual or consecutive basis. Rather, complex combinations are employed which are unique to the carers' particular circumstances. There is no strict criteria to guide the choice of strategies and, whilst consistency is important, most having a dominant mode of management, flexible access to a range of strategies is more effective than reliance upon a singular response. Receptiveness to new possibilities, along with the ability to create a sense of meaning out of what is demanded, are essential if carers are to achieve and retain a sense of personal control over their situation.

Organisation of time

> like I said, you've to organise and prioritise your time... my time was a precious resource not to be wasted. (Mrs Brown)

Time was identified as a crucial variable in the interface between the carers' occupational and domestic lives, requiring careful management. Active initiators, carers appraise the organisation and allocation of their time and, having pinpointed areas of concern, organise it so as to minimise wastage. For example, they get up earlier (often before 6 a.m.) and retire to bed later (often after midnight). The extra hours created enables them to carry out essential preparatory work. Distinguishing the more expendable components of their schedule, carers redefine their personal needs, limiting the time they devote to the pursuit of outside interests and to maintaining friendships which may have previously formed the mainstay of their social relationships. Non-work and non-caregiving activities are subordinated to rest and recuperation.

Carers also instigate modifications to their working lives; declining offers of overtime; arriving home more punctually; and, negotiating more suitable terms and conditions, for example, switching from full-time to part-time hours. Enabling them to meet time critical caregiving commitments, such changes are contingent upon the willingness of respective employers to make provision for a person's caring responsibilities and upon the degree of occupational discretion carers enjoy. In three cases, what may be termed work accommodation was instigated voluntarily, representing a positive decision on the carer's part to allocate a limited number of hours to employment. For one carer, such accommodation was involuntary, Mrs Smith complaining that she had no option other than to modify her employment activities.

Use of time

> it meant fittin' all the jobs in at odd times, erm, havin' to prepare everythin' again once you got home at night until such time as we got a freezer, shoppin' in the lunch hour an' tryin' to do all the washin' and not have it hanging about all over the show. (Mr Davies)

Closely tied in with the organisation of time, carers devise strategies which enable them to use their time constructively and effectively. For instance, they juggle two, sometimes three, spheres simultaneously, carry out domestic chores at unconventional hours and effectively utilise their lunch break. Lunch breaks are spent shopping, dealing with social service-related queries and attending to financial and legal matters. Those living near to their place of employment sometimes go home to attend to preparatory work. Alternatively, lunch breaks are sacrificed, carers working more intensively to expiate for lost time and to keep on or ahead of schedules. Keeping one step ahead is an important theme running through the narratives. This is only possible when time is utilised effectively.

As management strategies, the organisation and use of time are subject to constant review, this being initiated by an appraisal process in which carers take stock of how they consider themselves to be performing.

Securing a framework of support

Recognising the importance of involving others, carers enlist various types of assistance in the quest to negotiate their responsibilities. The first point of reference, whether seeking to acquire supervisory help or practical assistance, is immediate family, carers relying exclusively upon relatives during the early stages to monitor the dependant in their absence. As the person with dementia's condition deteriorates, a rota system is devised to ensure that he/she is never left unattended for an appreciable length of time.

In practice, support from kin is supplemented with various types of formal provision, carers enlisting the assistance of the day care, home help and district nursing services as well as the voluntary based Crossroads care attendant scheme. The amount and content of assistance varies from case to case.

Critical evaluation of support

This task requires the setting of operational standards based on the carers' understanding of what they need to supplement their coping skills and make their schedule work. These can be summarised as:

- flexibility
- accessibility
- comprehensiveness
- promptitude/reliability
- organizational sensitivity
- service responsiveness.

They are similar in many respects to the categories developed by others writing within the field of social care, for example, Huxley *et al.* (1990). Serving as yardsticks against which the effectiveness of provision will be gauged, they provide useful pointers for policy and practice. It is impossible to place them into some kind of priority order as there is a sense in which all are inseparable and should be seen as a complete package.

Operational standards

A key requirement of support is that it is flexible, accommodating the timing and practical requirements of schedules. Accessibility is a further requisite of effective provision, carers stipulating that support must be geographically accessible, i.e. locally based, and bureaucratically accessible, i.e. straightforward to negotiate and subject to minimal delays.

Comprehensiveness is described in terms of the range of care options available and their scope. Carers specify the need for an extensive range of household, personal care and sitting services, the amount and combination being at their discretion. Having identified time as a key issue in their occupational and domestic lives, they see promptitude and reliability as essential in any type of assistance, especially that intended to substitute for their presence.

Carers uphold that provision should not only respond with flexibility but also with sensitivity, stipulating that supporters must be sensitised to the carer's role as employees, to the dynamics of schedule management, to the perceived needs of the younger person with dementia and to the specific mix of difficulty they face.

The defining feature of responsive service provision is that it recognises the individuality of need, tailoring support to carers' schedule requirements, viewing their needs in a holistic rather than fragmented context and appreciating the temporal dynamics of the carer's task.

Having discerned carers' modest requirements, the chapter moves on to look at service response and suggestions are made to inform practical guidance. Comparisons between statutory and non-statutory services clearly depend on the availability of services in a particular area but point to the need to examine the relationship between needs and service response in district localities. During the course of evaluation it is intended to provide broad practical guidance rather than a comprehensive compendium of everything that should be done to support employed caregivers.

Flexibility

With respect to flexibility, statutory interventions do not fare well in this study. There appear to be discrepancies between the availability of support and the schedule requirements of employed carers.

Failing to accommodate the rhythm of their working day, carers are especially critical of statutory day care provision available. Whilst holding great potential for the support of employed carers, the reality of its impact is limited. The truncated day, contemptuously described as 'little more than a luncheon club', gives rise to problems of temporal accessibility:

> They're not open till half way through the morning and when you're workin' you need that bit of flexibility. It should be open by eight. (Mrs Brown)

Whilst the limited hours of availability (10.30 a.m. until 3.30 p.m.) may be appropriate to older carers, they are of little use to carers with employment commitments, especially full-time commitments. A priority area for improvement, carers require services which are available at times wide enough to accommodate the time requirements of their schedules, for instance, day care services which take their relative from early morning through until early evening.

In this study, support from Crossroads care attendants and immediate family fares more favourably in the carers' estimations. Sensitive to the time requirements of schedules, carers are able to control the timing of voluntary assistance which operates on a 24-hour basis seven days a week.

With respect to the practical requirements of schedules, the home help and district nursing services did not appear to meet requirements. Whilst relevant to the practical dimension of caregiving and able to counter enforced reductions in standards of domestic cleanliness, the restricted nature of tasks performed by home helps in the study area is problematic. Similarly, much of the potential of the district nursing service hinges on the provision of assistance with routine maintenance tasks. However, pressures on time militate against the performance of such tasks, priority being accorded to technical nursing procedures. Whilst theoretically available, routine assistance is provided on a sporadic basis, thereby failing to facilitate carers' practical requirements and limiting the relevance of the service.

In contrast, the Crossroads home respite scheme is clearly and specifically focused on relieving carers and prioritising their requirements. Embracing a mixture of personal care and sitting services, the diversity of tasks performed serve as an indicator of the potential relevance of such schemes in responding to the practical needs of employed caregivers and others.

Accessibility

In this sample day care services are geographically inaccessible. Considerable journeys of both distance (up to 28 miles) and time (up to 45 minutes) are made by two carers who, exasperated by the unpredictability of transport, resort to chauffeuring their husbands to the respective venues. Problems of accessibility are not confined to geography. Cumbrous procedures and lengthy delays in securing statutory support give rise to problems of bureaucratic accessibility, carers having limited time and energies to press for what they require.

Comprehensiveness

Not one form of provision was judged to be sufficiently comprehensive; criticisms centring upon the meagreness of allocations and the limited range of care options available.

Day care allocations of between one and three days per week are insufficient when struggling to hold down a full-time job, as are weekly or twice-weekly visits from the home help/district nurse. To be of optimum use, carers need assistance on each day they are required to work, weekends inclusive. Denouncing the assignment of day care places as biased towards meeting the needs of older carers, Mr Davies captures the consensus of opinion:

> It's all done for the oldies and that's no disrespect. They just think as they can't cope. Me, I'd to fight for the one day and nobody seemed to think how I managed with her and the job. Us younger people have different responsibilities to consider. (Mr Davies)

The inadequate level of day care provision prompted two carers to transfer to part-time hours and was sufficiently serious to be implicated in their decision to leave employment.

Having commended the support offered by Crossroads, carers recognise that its contribution is inevitably limited and that it is incapable of meeting demands on the scale required. Acknowledging the volunteer status of attendants, they do not wish to appear rapacious by requesting more than their 'fair share'.

Drawing attention to the limited range of care options available and to the importance of exercising choice when making arrangements, carers identified a number of shortfalls in provision. The scope for improvement is considerable, priorities being: to devise interventions specifically for younger people with dementia and their supporters; to develop an extensive range of household, personal care and sitting services which reflect the diversity of need and which are available at times wide enough to accommodate the requirements of schedules; to develop supplementary care arrangements to assist carers to negotiate their commitments in the event of short-term contingencies.

Promptness and reliability

Voluntary provision in the study area is prompt and reliable. In contrast, there is little sense of a reliable alliance between carers and statutory providers. Deviations from prearranged appointment times, along with last-minute cancellations, pose logistical difficulties for employed carers whose schedules, whilst sufficiently flexible to accommodate minor discrepancies, are thrown into disarray by persistently late and unreliable services. Deliberating upon the intricacies of rescheduling, carers uphold that by committing such acts supporters are, in effect, devaluing their work, presuming they can easily adjust their schedules. Once again day care figures prominently in the carers' critical commentaries, the perennial problem of transport being identified as one of its most frustrating aspects. Carers are emphatic in their insistence that day care should be serviced by prompt and utterly reliable transportation. However, reports of three-hour delays are not uncommon and, on occasion, transport fails to arrive. Whilst waiting, dependants often become agitated, compounding the carers' frustrations:

> he'd be pacing the floor and he'd start throwin' anything in sight... See, he wasn't a frail old man who needed a stick, he was very strong and sometimes he'd be tryin' to undress himself and getting frustrated because he couldn't remember how. He'd often need a change of clothes before he'd even got in the car. Had he been elderly he mighten have been so bad. (Mrs Smith)

Problems of transport have been repeatedly identified in studies of day care and it remains unclear as to whether they are resolvable. Indications are that when the matter is given priority an improved service can be provided.

Whilst generally prompt, informal assistance is unreliable as a means of long-term support, carers drawing attention to the difficulties of ensuring continuity of provision over time. Beset by life's vicissitudes, the circumstances of family members change, prompting them to reappraise their priorities and subsequently influencing their capacity and willingness to provide help. Depending upon their nature, changes have a range of consequences from the scaling down of activities to the withdrawal of assistance.

Organisational sensitivity

Once again, statutory interventions do not fare well, health and social care professionals being reported to display an attitude of indifference towards the carers' roles as employees in the wider society, remaining nonchalant to the dynamics of schedule management and failing to respond with sensitivity to the perspective of the person with younger onset dementia. As the first-hand accounts reveal, organisational insensitivity results in distress for carers and their relatives.

The most consistent need, spontaneously expressed by carers, is recognition as a distinct client group, requiring a complement of specialist, age-sensitive interventions which preserve the dignity and self-respect of their relative and which take account of their lifestyle:

> They don't seem to realise as its a whole different ball game when it catches them in their prime and as a carer you're different as well. You've nothin' in common with the golden oldie brigade because you're still at work and maybe still have kiddies. As things stand at the moment, they add to your heartache an' it's high time someone realised as we need services geared towards younger ones. (Mr Davies)

Statutory provision, most notably day care, fails to meet this fundamental need and carers are dovetailed into services designed primarily for older people. Falling between the criteria for older people and adult services they are, in Mulligan's (1994, p.23) terms, 'out of place and out of time'.

Once more carers express reservations over statutory day care. An important, albeit problematic form of respite provision, it is judged to be unsatisfactory on a number of grounds. First, relatives lack suitable outlets for their recreational interests:

> It wasn't designed for people like [husband]... They'd sit talking about the great war, well, he wasn't around then. What was the use of that? ... I remember one occasion droppin' him off an' the woman shouts 'Come on, we're makin' Easter bonnets today' and I thought my God this is awful. He should'a been in the fresh air or something, anything but that. (Mrs Smith)

Age-sensitive therapies and diversional activities are judged to be of the essence if the individual's competencies are to be sustained and their quality of life preserved. Describing their relative's expressed dislike of older people's day care and their distress at attending a centre where older, physically incapacitated members are present, carers call for specialist facilities to be established for and offered exclusively to younger people with dementia. Consistent with previous accounts (Quinn 1996), this constitutes a priority area for improvement.

Second, day care staff spend a disproportionate amount of their time meeting the dependency needs of frail attenders, subsequently neglecting to accommodate the younger person's greater degree of physical strength. Young and active, Mr Brown and Mr Smith had both left the day centre unaccompanied, raising concerns as to their safety whilst their wives were out working.

Onset at an early, active stage of life has the effect of accentuating problematic behaviours, a factor warranting close consideration when devising suitable care programmes. Carers voiced concern that professionals had overlooked this matter and described how their relatives' disruptive influence posed a threat to frail older people. Staff training and level of staffing appeared to reflect a lack of awareness of this group's particular needs.

Due in part to the above limitations, carers are reluctant to enlist formal assistance and express ambivalence at having to resort to inappropriate services:

> To see a good man go down hill and be robbed of his future, spendin' his days with a bunch of old folk, it's very sad. I couldn't have managed to work without him goin' but it's awful to think he's winded up there. I defy anyone to come to terms with it. Had they put him with people his own age it may have been easier. (Mrs Brown)

> She's my mum and she's only in her 40s and it just kills me to think of her sat with oldies more than twice her age… OK, it lets me do my voluntary work but it also adds to my problems in other ways, erm, emotionally speaking. (Mrs Crosby)

Knowing the respective covering arrangements are not a positive experience for the person with dementia adds to the carers' distress.

Voluntary provision provided through the Crossroads care attendant scheme responds with sensitivity to the needs of the younger person with dementia and their carers. Non-stigmatising, relatives are able to pursue their preferred activities and are respected as individuals. Continuity of helper is highly valued as it facilitates the establishment of relationships. Carers feel secure in the knowledge that whilst at work their relative is in the charge of a competent person and that the break is a positive experience for him or her. Making a distinctive contribution, Crossroads care attendants respect the ways in which carers define their problems and are sensitive to the respite function which employment provides.

Service responsiveness

In the study area, statutory interventions, such as day care and home help services, fail to recognise the individuality of need and neglect to incorporate carers' temporal and practical requirements into service priorities. Internal service considerations appear to take precedence as carers are dragooned into pre-existing menus of provision without due regard for their specific circumstances. Failing to rise to the challenge of recent legislation, individually tailored packages of care are non-existent and there is no evidence of service providers seeking out innovative ways to overcome some of the specific constellations of difficulty carers face. Voluntary provision (Crossroads), in contrast, is tailored to suit each family situation. Unambiguously provided for carers, supporters acquaint themselves with individual structures for coping and are judged to be attentive to the needs of employed carers.

Having detailed how carers set about negotiating their commitments on a daily basis, attention now turns to a consideration of how they manage in the situational context of an emergency.

Crisis modes of coping – contingency plans

Incorporated within schedules are contingency plans, designed to assist carers negotiate their responsibilities in the event of a crisis. Crises include situations where the usual covering arrangements fall through due to unforeseen circumstances. As with schedule development, levels of preparedness varied. Exercising foresight, Mrs Brown and Mrs Smith made provisions for potential difficulties when first devising their schedules. In contrast, Mrs Crosby and Mr Davies learned from experience, formulating contingency plans after having been engulfed by a series of crises.

By definition, crises generate practical needs, demand immediate responses and have the potential to cause considerable disruption and distress both at work and at home. The aim in devising contingency plans is to minimise disruption and distress and to ensure sufficient flexibility in responding to situations as they unfold. Competent adaptors, carers cope actively with setbacks, securing short-term help and/or adapting their employment commitments until the usual arrangements can be resumed. Leaves of absence are taken, holiday entitlements used and, in extreme cases, carers take illegitimate days off work. Should the crisis persist for any length of time, the entire covering arrangements are reappraised.

Temporal aspects of the management experience

Based on the transactional model of stress, which acknowledges the dynamic nature of caregiving and the fluidity of coping responses, it is useful to explore the time aspects of the carers' management experience. A model comprising five graduated stages is proposed. It shows how the task of nego-tiating the demands of caregiving and employment is not resolved at a single point in time but rather by a continuing process of response to the changing conditions under which carers operate and to the success or failure of their coping efforts. Key transition points are identified which serve as markers, signposting the types of assistance most useful at a given point.

Stage 1: Managing uncertainty

During the early days, carers encounter a series of problems, mostly minor, which they overcome by exercising a modicum of common sense. For exam-ple, Mrs Crosby and Mr Davies left sufficient provisions for their relatives who experienced difficulties in preparing their own meals. Similarly, Mrs Brown and Mrs Smith, whose spouses remained in employment, ensured that their husbands and their husbands' work colleagues had a contact number should anything untoward occur. At the same time, tactful efforts were made to persuade them to leave work. A distinctive issue specific to carers of youn-ger people with dementia, attempts to persuade relatives to leave employment are met with resistance. Whilst experiencing difficulties in per-forming organisational and administrative duties, relatives continue to assign importance to their work role and are reluctant to relinquish it.

Providing intermittent assistance with the activities of daily living to a relative who may or may not have received a confirmed diagnosis of Alzhei-mer's disease, carers have little sense of how onerous their commitment may prove to be. Frustrated by the medical profession's reluctance to diagnose dementia at an early age, the context is a pervasive sense of not knowing.

Structures for coping have yet to be formulated. Formal provision is non-existent. Aside from counselling and information support it would prove intrusive. With little or no background experience, carers display a good deal of initial innocence. The transition to Stage 2 is marked by a sense of accumulating responsibility and the imposition of constraints on carers' time.

Stage 2: Trial and error

Carers continue to provide intermittent assistance to their relative whose confusion and memory impairment is sufficiently pronounced to preclude their involvement in paid employment. Interval dependence – that is, how long relatives can be left without some form of supervision – enters the frame. Aware of the potential risks if left to their own devices, carers are reluctant to leave their relative for an appreciable length of time. Relatives usually remain physically robust and carers try to prevent them from engaging in activities which might threaten their well being, to find suitable outlets for their energies and to minimise their awareness of their diminishing abilities.

It was at this stage that Mrs Brown and Mrs Smith began to contemplate the practicalities of dependence, formulating tentative schedules to assist them negotiate their accumulating responsibilities. In contrast, Mrs Crosby and Mr Davies maintained a facade of normality and tried to succeed in spite of a lack of organisation.

Schedule formulation is characterised by a good deal of trial and error and it is possible to see two distinct approaches. The first is somewhat 'hit and miss', carers trying out one strategy after another, whilst the second is more thoughtful and methodical. Whilst increasingly able to appreciate discrete aspects of the situation, carers operate with a degree of residual uncertainty, describing this stage in terms of 'finding one's bearings' (Mrs Brown). Reluctant to access formal support, they rely exclusively upon informal supporters to provide a monitoring service. Aside from taking time off to accompany relatives to medical appointments, working hours remain unaltered. Preparatory work is undertaken during the evenings.

Carers progress to Stage 3 after acknowledging the reality of the situation, the importance of a proactive response and their inability to manage single-handedly.

Stage 3: Getting to grips

Acknowledging the challenge and appraising the adequacy of existing arrangements carers, by necessity, devise a way of coping and begin planning, albeit tentatively, for the future.

As the disease takes hold of relatives their safety becomes an all-consuming concern, carers responding to the increasingly precarious situation by attempting to secure supervisory care for the duration of their absence. A rota system is sometimes devised and supervision becomes a passive yet constant and vital aspect of the carers' workload.

Requiring a mixture of household and sitting services, carers reluctantly enlist support from formal channels. Responding proactively, they gradually begin to reorganise their time and initiate alterations to their working lives. Important compromise strategies, these alterations are designed to protect the carers' employment whilst simultaneously enabling them to assume a considerable degree of responsibility for their relative. Additionally, they begin to redefine their personal needs, curtailing outside interests.

In the constant attempts to maximise positive outcomes, carers test out various strategies, their successful implementation giving rise to personal satisfaction. Acquiring know-how, they are increasingly able to pigeonhole demands into various strategies, to mobilise resources and to exercise discretionary judgement.

The transition to Stage 4 is marked by a sense of being extended to the limit, by the constant need to adjust to the realities of the situation and by the need to mobilise more formal provision.

Stage 4: Establishing the upper hand

This stage is characterised by carers striving to maintain a semblance of orderliness and organisation in daily life. The all-encompassing demands on their time and energies, coupled with a sense of constant responsibility, are defining features, intermittent dependency in daily living having been succeeded by persistent dependency.

This continuous process of negotiation is often described as a juggling act and organisation and planning are essential in managing the increasingly complex timetables. Possessing an intuitive grasp of the situation and boasting a wealth of local knowledge, two carers established themselves as experts at this stage. Implementing a broad range of management strategies, carers fundamentally reorganise their time and ensure its optimal use. Whilst recognising the importance of looking after themselves, they once again redefine their personal needs, devoting less time to other relatives and to the maintenance of friendships. Outside interests are virtually non-existent. Direct relief of a number of household and personal care tasks, along with flexible sitting services, are required.

Having reached this stage, carers establish criteria for recognising when they can no longer continue to negotiate their multiple commitments.

Exploring the rationale behind the decision to leave employment, the relative's age is identified as an important factor, carers maintaining that had they been older they would almost certainly persevere and remain at work. Whilst intellectually they know their relative will not survive indefinitely, his or her life expectancy is thought to be greater than that of an older person with the disease. Such is the pressure on carers at this stage that they commonly terminate their employment.

Stage 5: Keeping going

The final stage is characterised by carers striving to make the best of their circumstances.

Having reached a point where they perceived that it was in the interests of neither party to maintain the caregiving arrangements, Mr Davies and Mrs Smith admitted their spouses into permanent care. Whilst the period of direct caregiving was ended, entry into care did not signal the end of caregiving. Other forms of care, namely, preservative, (re)constructive and reciprocal (Nolan, Keady and Grant 1995), continued as carers shifted their responsibilities and took on an active role in ensuring that professionals had the relevant information to provide good care. Both took steps to create a new beginning for themselves, Mrs Smith returning to part-time employment and Mr Davies actively seeking work. Whilst seemingly ill-prepared, professionals withdrew their support, assuming that carers were able to 'stand back on the old two feet' (Mr Davies). As with the first stage, the context is one of uncertainty. Mrs Brown and Mrs Crosby continued to look after their relatives and attempted to come to terms with their non-employed status.

Practice implications

The model presented here is intended to serve as a sensitising device, representing and summarising a range of potentially important factors. It highlights the dynamic quality of the carers' experience and the changing nature of their support requirements. As demands are resolved and new ones emerge, different types and mixes of support are required. Interventions rejected as intrusive whilst managing uncertainty, for example, day care, often become fundamental to attempts to manage the situation later on. Therefore, it is essential that those professionals involved in assessing, commissioning and providing services see the management experience of the carer as an ongoing process with transition points and changing demands.

The model underscores the need for a flexible approach to assessment. Assigned new prominence as the cornerstone of effective provision (Carers (Recognition and Services) Act 1995), assessments should not be viewed as ends in themselves or as discrete, one-off events, but rather as the first stage in a process of continual monitoring and review. If interventions are to be tailored to situations as they unfold, an ongoing dialogue between carers and professionals is vital as is access to reassessment. Further, it is essential that due recognition is given to the carers' perspective and to their varying levels of expertise.

Attention is drawn to the importance of an early diagnosis and to the potential usefulness of age-appropriate information at key transition points. During the first and second stages information detailing the likely course and duration of the illness would enable carers to formulate a realistic picture of their likely future and to answer their queries regarding 'what can I expect next?' Similarly, information about local services and how these may be accessed would make the system less intimidating. Unfortunately, carers often appear to acquire disparate fragments of information in a piecemeal way.

Finally, the model highlights the importance of continuing to support carers once relatives have entered residential nursing home or hospital care. Carers require assistance to create a balanced perspective, to acknowledge the value of what they have achieved and to plan for the future.

Discussion

It is evident that current assessment and service provision often fails to meet the challenge laid down in legislation, that is, to provide a range of services which respond with flexibility and sensitivity to the assessed needs of individuals and their carers (DoH 1989). Professionals often fail to recognise the carers of younger people with dementia as a distinct group and services are frequently organised and delivered in ways which disregard the realities of their daily lives and add to their distress. The scope for improvement is considerable and it is hoped that the operational standards specified in this chapter will provide useful pointers for policy and practice. It is attention to these sorts of detail that will ensure the provision of high quality services which meet the needs of younger people with dementia and their employed caregivers. The experiences of the dementia services for younger people in the Merseyside region demonstrate that without significant additional resources it is possible for agencies to collaborate and to provide suitable support for this group (Alzheimer's Disease Society 1995).

Having described the difficulties carers encounter in their quest to negotiate their caregiving and employment responsibilities and having conveyed a sense of the ingenuity and resilience they display as they set about their daily lives, it is hoped that the chapter has provided insights which are instructive to employers, specifically the importance of compassionate and flexible responses to the dilemmas carers face. Caring is not a business relationship but an emotional one, and it is essential that carers are afforded flexible terms and conditions of employment. Piecemeal measures will no longer suffice and in future employers should be required to offer a menu of accessible policies which reflect the diversity of carers' needs. Given that change has been identified as an important feature of the intersection of caregiving and employment (Phillips 1995), it is essential that employers establish an ongoing dialogue with their caregiving employees and that policies are periodically reassessed to ensure their continuing responsiveness.

CHAPTER II

Young Carers

Individual Circumstances and Practice
Consideration in Dementia Caregiving

Jane Gilliard

Introduction

Between 1990 and 1996 I worked as a counsellor at a memory disorders
clinic in the south-west of England. My role was to provide support to the
carers of people who attended the clinic and who had been assessed as having some form of dementia. I contacted carers shortly after their relative first
attended for assessment and diagnosis, and remained in touch with them for
as long as the carer required support. Most of the people I saw during this
time were the spouses or adult children of people who had a diagnosis of
dementia. They probably ranged in age from early 40s to early 90s.

One day I was asked to see the carers of a 61-year-old man (Mr J), a wid-
ower, who was attending the clinic on a regular basis as part of a trial of a new
therapeutic agent. This man had seven children, most of whom were grown
up, married and living away from home. He was cared for by the youngest
two, aged 18 and 15 when we first met. It made me realise for the first time
that dementia is not just something that happens to older people. Its effects
'spread across the generations, like ripples in a pond' (see Gilliard 1996;
Tibbs 1995). The ripples also touched young people who, as part of a family,
were often overshadowed in the glare of support provision. This chapter,
therefore, will seek to explore the experience of young carers (that is, those
aged less than 21) and will use a case study approach to highlight service and
practice considerations. The chapter commences with the case study that
formed the basis of my exploratory work in this area (Gilliard 1996).

Case study: Mr J

My professional background is in social work, and at one time I carried a caseload which predominantly consisted of children and families. A few years later this experience stood me in good stead for working with young carers of people with dementia. Nevertheless, my previous experience of working with young people had been a while ago and I had to give careful consideration about how best to support this group. In dementia care there was no guidance for me about working with them, no guidance for the young people themselves and no books that explained dementia to young people in a straightforward and accessible manner. The only publication with which I was familiar was an Alzheimer's Disease Society (ADS) booklet aimed at explaining dementia to primary school aged children (Evans, undated).

I planned my first meeting with the carers of Mr J. I was asked particularly to see the younger one, a 15-year-old boy. The usual counselling setting of two chairs not quite facing each other, and two people talking for about an hour seemed much too formal and threatening to offer to a 15 year old. We needed something that was more relaxed, where we could begin to develop a relationship in which he could learn to trust me. At our first meeting I suggested we go to a nearby cafe. I invited him to tell me about himself, his interests, his school and his plans for the future. Sometimes he talked about his father for a short while, and then the conversation moved back to him. I decided not to push him too much at this first meeting.

The next time we met we went for a walk. This allowed the opportunity for beginning to confront some of the issues. Silence is more tolerable when you're walking alongside someone, so we could choose to talk or not as we walked. Eye contact can be avoided, so one can tackle some of the meatier issues without having to look at the person you're talking to. In some ways this almost gives a sense of anonymity. There were distractions, so we could escape from confronting the issues by stopping to watch some small children feeding the ducks or to look at the birds. In short, having an activity as a focus in which we could still talk about all sorts of things including his father's condition, provided the sort of safe environment to make a start.

At about this time I had started writing a book to explain dementia to young people (Gilliard 1995). I wanted the book to address the issues which young carers needed to have answered. I discussed its content with the young carer with whom I had been working. I asked his advice on what topics we should cover and started by asking, 'What do young people in your situation want to know?' This approach began to open up other areas for us to discuss and it became an opportunity to invite and encourage the young person to talk without seeming to be confrontational. In the event, it was almost as if we were talking about the problems that other people would have, distancing the ownership of the myriad concerns and problems.

Finally we moved on to 'heavier' issues. A local school had produced some artwork for the book and I invited the young carer to help me select the pictures that should be used in its final publication. We spent a morning looking at these pictures and discussing what they meant to us. We talked about whether they projected a positive or negative image of dementia and of caring, and considered which he liked and, more importantly, why. We also talked about the images he found uncomfortable. Through this collaborative and inclusive approach, we were able to use the pictures as a base from which we could move to talk about his personal caring situation. Again, we didn't have to have eye contact – we were on our knees poring over the pictures that were spread over the floor. We could have silences while we looked at the pictures, without feeling uncomfortable. We could have diversions and change the subject without any discomfort.

Practice issues

Counselling carers of people with dementia can involve a person-centred approach (Egan 1990), i.e. the starting point should be with the person being offered counselling and we meet them 'where they're at'. Working with young carers is no different, although it does require careful consideration and preparation. Moreover, the counselling relationship does break some of the rules – probably the most obvious being the importance of eye contact. My experience has certainly been that the formal 'let's sit and talk' approach achieves little with young people. More appropriate methods appear to be to 'get alongside' the young person by engaging in some form of activity, and allowing the young person to talk when they are ready, within the confines of that activity. There may be times when they want to talk in some depth and we should be ready to sit and listen. Building an initial relationship on trust appears much more significant with young carers, and I have listed below some suggestions in forming this relationship.

- Do not rush. Do not expect a young person to open up to you at your first meeting.

- Engage in an activity in which they can feel safe to remain silent and to avoid eye contact.

- Do not feel that you have to talk about their 'problems' all the time.

- Use props to stimulate discussion. Talking about the pictures for the book was probably the most productive session I had with my young carer. I could have asked him to be the artist, or we could have used other media to open our discussion.

- It may sometimes be helpful to talk about the issues in the third person, as when the young carer told me what issues he thought other young people would want addressed in the book.

It is important to remember that the counsellor/supporter may not be the only person who is trying to support a young carer. They may be in touch with support services through their school, or they may have a favourite relative or friend in whom they prefer to confide. It is possible that the professional role should be to inform that supporter about dementia so that they are best placed to help the young carer. I am not advocating a breach of confidentiality involving the personal circumstances, but rather a general discussion about what dementia means for people with dementia and their family. In the case of the young carer, I talked to the school counsellor, the head of year at school and to the social worker from the local area team. I explained to them what dementia is and how it impacts on all those involved. It then seemed more appropriate for the young carer to be supported by the school services with which he already had regular daily contact.

We have to beware of making assumptions about what is best. There were two young carers in this family and my work with the older child was quite different from that of the younger. The older child was emotionally more mature and we had regular 'chatting' sessions over a cup of tea sitting at her kitchen table. I suggested to her that she might find a support group helpful, and was able to give her details of two existing groups in her local area. One was a support group for young carers. Newly established, it was attended by several young people who were caring for relatives with a number of different conditions. The support group organised a variety of activities, many of which were simply fun and to give the young people a break. The other group was for carers of people with dementia. They were mostly older people, although there were a small number of adult–child carers. The young carer chose to go to this group. She wanted to mix with people whose relative had the same as her father, even though she was probably about 40 years younger than most of the others. By attending the group, however, she learnt and shared a lot. She listened to their experiences and they supported her. They became almost like a substitute family for her.

A personal reflection

As I reflected on my work with this family, and with others, it occurred to me that, although there may be relatively few young people who are the main carers for a relative with dementia, there are a number of others who are affected by having a relative in the extended family with dementia. There was one family, for example, who had always lived with their grandmother. She now had dementia and became very disturbed, often threatening her granddaughters, sometimes with violence. It reached a critical point at which the girls were judged to be at risk, and their grandmother had to be removed from the home for their safety. The impact of this move on the grandmother, her daughter and her granddaughters was immense.

Another family had decided to move grandmother in with them when they felt she was no longer safe to live on her own. This meant that the children had to change bedrooms, and two of them had to share a room for the first time. The older child became resentful and difficult. Her parents began to have to deal with behaviour problems from her for the first time.

I was often asked for advice on how to explain the condition to children or grandchildren. It seemed especially hard on a young person who is experiencing all the turmoil of adolescence to have to deal with the added stress of a relative with dementia. It happened at a time when they don't want to be seen to be different from their peers. It is very hard to own up to having a relative with dementia when your friends probably don't understand the condition. The young person is then labelled as the one with the 'loony' dad or granddad.

Much has been written about the impact of dementia on carers (e.g. Taylor 1987), but little about young people as carers. From my experience, they share similar emotions and turmoil, but there are additional challenges, mostly associated with the other stresses and changes that are happening in their lives. They may well feel sad. The personality changes associated with dementia mean that they, too, have 'lost' a relative. They may want to be involved in the caring, or they may want to shut the person with dementia away. Either way, they are as liable to feel guilty about their relationship with the person as any other more formally recognised carer. Young people may be prone to mood swings, so they may become more easily angry or frustrated. I have heard of one young carer, for example, who turned to petty crime as a way of expressing her emotions during this difficult time.

They may feel embarrassed. It may be difficult to own that you have a relative with dementia. They may feel that they cannot invite their friends round to the house, and then they begin to become socially isolated from their peer group. They may feel that they don't want to be seen with their relative. This can be especially difficult if the person with dementia is a parent because there are occasions when one is expected to be seen with one's parent – the end-of-term concert, or school parent's evening, for example.

They may become worried about 'inheriting' dementia and will need a great deal of reassurance and support about this issue. Their fears may develop out of all proportion. Teenage children often live in a very black and white world, in which feelings become over-exaggerated.

In caring for a person with dementia, there is often a role transition. Wives have to take over the jobs that their husband has always done. Children have to become the parents to their own parents. In my experience, this can be one of the hardest adjustments for any child carer to make, regardless of their age. To have to do the things for your parent that you have always relied on and expected them to do for you is very hard to accept. If you are only young, it may be even harder. It isn't always easy for the person with dementia, either. The 61-year-old man, whose family I described earlier, has talked to me about how difficult it is for him to watch his daughter taking responsibility for managing the household accounts, for example. He used to run his own business, and it reduced him to tears to have to rely on his teenage daughter in this way.

Young carers will feel angry and may blame the person with dementia. If they are not the main carer, it may be that the person with dementia is taking up much of their parents' time, so that the young person feels shut out. Or they may have lost their valued privacy, as in the case of the granddaughter who had to share a bedroom with her sister. The anger may be projected in all directions – possibly at the person with dementia, or other relatives, parents or siblings, at school, in the community, with God. 'It's not fair!' is often the rallying cry of children and young people. They should be encouraged to talk about their feelings. They should be told how they can help their family, how they can communicate with their relative who has dementia.

Conclusion

This chapter has attempted to demonstrate, through a practical and anecdotal approach, that dementia can affect young people, although this is often overlooked in service planning and delivery. Young people may be the children, grandchildren, nephews, nieces or neighbours of a person with dementia. They may be the main carer, although they are more likely to be in the circle of secondary carers or significant others (Gilliard 1996).

The needs of young people as carers should not be ignored. They experience the double pressures of passing through one of the most turbulent times during the life course, at the same time as being the carer of a person with dementia. I have attempted through case illustration to give some suggestions of ways to make support to young people accessible. This is not intended to be a definitive or prescriptive list of ideas. It is meant to act as a springboard for innovation in professional practice when working with young carers of people with dementia.

CHAPTER 12

Family Caregiving and Younger People with Dementia

Dynamics, Experiences and Service Expectations

John Keady and Mike Nolan

What a waste of my husband's life. What a sorry, sorry waste of his life.

Introduction

Those heartfelt words were spoken by a carer when reflecting upon the death of her husband from Alzheimer's disease at the age of 56 years; he had been diagnosed some three years earlier and for the final two years of his life had lived in a nursing home in North Wales. However, despite the above stark image of dementia we feel it is important to develop a better understanding of the changing nature of care over time, which reflects both positive and negative aspects. By listening to the accounts of bereaved spouses of younger people with dementia, we were struck by the emotional power of these narratives, with a broad range of experience being crammed into a few years. Moreover, and as we shall discuss later, the death of the younger person with dementia was not, of itself, a release from the emotional impact of caregiving; indeed if anything, for some spouse carers (and their children) the stressors actually increased with the fear of genetic transmission of dementia (particularly Alzheimer's disease) and a heightened sensitivity to the changes brought about by its onset and progression. So, for example, one carer in the study constantly checked that their memory was still intact for fear of 'getting it [dementia] as well'. Identifying significant issues and intervening in these circumstances requires a skilled understanding of family needs support that continues long after the death of a partner.

Reflecting the above, this chapter is about the dynamics, experiences and service expectations of carers of younger people with dementia. As such it complements the previous two in this section by Diane Seddon (Chapter 10) and Jane Gilliard (Chapter 11), and although there may be some overlap between these accounts, this is important as it further validates the processes that exist and helps to identify common threads. However, to minimise any unnecessary replication, this chapter will not explore fully the coping strategies over the continuum of care as these have already been rehearsed by Diane Seddon in Chapter 10. Rather, we will draw upon the experiences of 22 family carers of younger people with dementia in order to present an overview of their service experiences at different points. These experiences will be framed within a temporal model of care (see Keady and Nolan 1993; Nolan, Grant and Keady 1996) to help contextualise caregiving, from the subtle early adjustment at the first changes in dementia through to the experience of bereavement itself. The framework for this exploration consists of six stages, or transition points, as follows:

1. Building on the Past

2. Recognising the Need

3. Taking It On

4. Working Through It

5. Reaching the End

6. A New Beginning.

It is important, however, to point out that we do not see these stages as a rigid framework intended to mask the individual experience of carers. Rather they are a device to aid thinking, to raise awareness of some shared aspects of caregiving and to sensitise practitioners to a number of issues likely to be relevant to their assessment and intervention models.

In order to set the scene the chapter will begin with a brief review of the literature on studies which have explored the service expectations and needs of younger people with dementia and their carers. The study methodology and sample will then be described followed by an overview of caring using the six-stage model of care. Where appropriate each of these transition points and experiences will be supported by quotations, and practice implications will be outlined towards the end of the chapter.

Whilst we attempt to capture the lived experience of caring in dementia, it is important to highlight a limitation of the study in that we did not interview younger people with dementia about their own experiences and service expectations. Such an account is vital if a more complete picture is to be obtained. Data we have collected from people with dementia themselves has been drawn predominantly from an older population, although it did include the contribution from one person with Alzheimer's disease who was aged 67 years (see Keady and Gilliard in press; Keady and Bender 1998; Keady and Nolan 1995a, 1995b; Keady, Nolan and Gilliard 1995). However, to compensate for some of the deficits in our own data, we will briefly rehearse the subjective accounts provided in two published works by Davis (1989) and McGowin (1993), as the voices of younger people with dementia are ones which need to be more clearly articulated.

Experiencing dementia

In the last ten years two books, both emanating from the USA, have been written by younger people with Alzheimer's disease (Davis 1989; McGowin 1993). The first, that by the Reverend Robert Davis, provided important insights into the subjective experience of Alzheimer's disease. The author was a church pastor and he graphically portrayed his journey into Alzheimer's disease, and the impact that this had upon all aspects of his life. The full gauntlet of human emotions featured in this account, in particular the anger and frustration experienced during early adjustment and later in his quest for an explanation of his cumulative losses. During his account Davis described dementia as a 'dark veil that only very occasionally lifted' (Davis 1989, p.63) and detailed how he required the unflinching support of his wife, his own spiritual faith and the eventual knowledge of the diagnosis before he could gradually come to terms with the full meaning of Alzheimer's disease.

Diana Friel McGowin, who was aged 45 at the time of her account, also provided a powerful description of her experience of Alzheimer's disease and the huge disruption to work and family life that this caused. In direct contrast to the experience of the Reverend Robert Davis, McGowin's partner initially took the brunt of her displaced anger, a situation exacerbated by her husband's refusal to acknowledge any significant changes in either her emotions or behaviour, and his firm belief that 'things would get back to normal' as time progressed. For carers, this attempt to 'normalise events' is not an unusual occurrence (see Clarke 1995). Indeed, a qualitative study conducted by Garwick, Detzner and Boss (1994), which used a symbolic interactionist approach to analyse the verbal experience of 38 families caring during the early stages of Alzheimer's disease, contended that it was usual for family members to adapt to an uncertain stressor(s) by ignoring, or denying, their very existence. By using this strategy established roles can be preserved and routines can continue 'as normal', a strategy McGowin herself recognises towards the end of her book:

> My most troublesome fears revolve around the same theme. Would my husband of over twenty years protect and take care of me should I decline further? He is a stalwart, a stoic, and we had only recently regained a state of grace in our marriage, after many troubled years. (1993, p.114)

It is also interesting that McGowin recognises the need for protection and future care, but that professional interventions to plan for such events are mentioned rarely in these exchanges.

Despite a wealth of studies in the last 20 years exploring the nature of stress, coping and service experiences of carers of people with dementia (for key texts and literature reviews see Knight, Lutzky and Macofsky-Urban 1993; Kuhlman *et al.* 1991; Vitaliano, Young and Russo 1991; Woods 1995) such limitations persist for carers of people with dementia at all ages. However, in the UK at least, it was not until the turn of this decade that the needs of younger people with dementia and their family carers began to figure more prominently in policy and practice debates. A major step towards this greater recognition was taken in 1991 when the Alzheimer's Disease Society (ADS) took up the campaign by carers in the Mersey Region Health Authority and published their six-point *Declaration of Rights for Younger People with Dementia and their Carers* (ADS 1991). This Declaration of Rights called for:

1. Fully informed medical assessment

2. Recognition of the need for specialist services

3. Support following diagnosis, to include:

    *   specialist day care services
    *   appropriate residential care
    *   implementation of care management

4. Access to welfare benefits

5. Retrospective reinstatement of rights and benefits

6. Appropriate training and support.

In 1992 this Declaration of Rights was included in a follow-up information pamphlet produced by the ADS which focused on the younger person with dementia (ADS 1992b), and heralded the start of an annual national conference to explore issues for younger people with dementia and their family carers. Nineteen-ninety-one also saw the publication of an innovative planning report by Cox (1991) at the Dementia Services Development Centre in Stirling, Scotland, which highlighted issues that service planners and providers should take into account when responding to 'pre-senile dementia'. Updated in 1994 (Cox and McLennan 1994) this publication continues to present an accessible overview of some of the more telling experiences of younger people with dementia and their family carers, such as: increased financial loss and disruption; the impact of dementia on adolescents; the affect on social networks; the pronounced physical activity of the younger person with dementia. On this latter point, Keady and Nolan (1997) summarised these experiences as involving heightened:

- physical behaviour, including aggression
- restlessness
- expressions of frustration
- levels of awareness
- expressions of fear
- feelings of distress
- disruption
- unpredictability
- sleeplessness.

Naturally, the presence of such behaviours, either individually or collectively, can increase family stress immeasurably, necessitating active community intervention, which may well include admission into local care services. Similar findings have been reported in small-scale qualitative studies focusing on the family carer's subjective interpretation of their experience (ADS 1995; Cox 1991; Cox and McLennan 1994; Dementia Relief Trust 1996; Furst and Sperlinger 1992; Keady and Nolan 1994; Sperlinger and Furst 1994; Williams, Keady and Nolan 1995).

In order for improvements to occur, Keady and Nolan (1997) identified three principal needs for family carers of younger people with dementia: first, the need for dedicated and flexible services; second, compensation for financial hardship and loss; third, extension to the role of the dementia care practitioner. On this latter point a recent detailed study by Ferran *et al.* (1996) in Merseyside suggested that there was a need for a specialised multidisciplinary service for younger people with dementia and their carers, both in terms of diagnosis and support, a suggestion which is highly relevant but elusive to realise.

Methodology

The section which follows is based on an interview study conducted by the main author. Data were collected during in-depth semistructured interviews with 58 family carers of people with dementia, of which 18 were caring for a younger person with dementia at home. This sample included 12 co-habitant spouses: age range 47–64 years; caring history 1 year–8 years: mean = 5.2 years and 6 adult children: age range 21–39 years; caring history 6 months–7 years: mean = 4.1 years. Of the six adult child carers, four cared for their parent at a distance, and two had moved in with their parent to provide more full-time support. Four further spouse carers in the sample had previously cared for a younger person with dementia, but no longer did so owing either to the death of that person ($n=2$) or their admission into nursing home care ($n=2$). The data collected were analysed from a grounded theory perspective using constant comparative analysis (Glaser 1978; Glaser and Strauss 1967) in order to build a better understanding of the experience of dementia. All interviews took place in the carer's home and were tape recorded and transcribed by hand on the day of the interview. The interviews were completed in Wales and North West England between 1992 and 1996 and entry into the study depended upon a diagnosis of dementia by a consultant psychiatrist using DSM-III-R (American Psychiatric Association 1987) or DSM-IV-R criteria (American Psychiatric Association 1994) depending upon the year of interview. The semi-structured interview schedule began with an open discussion of the carer's transition into care and experience of caring. Coping strategies and support networks were also discussed together with carers' experiences of support from statutory and voluntary services. In the more structured part of the interview, Nolan and Grant's (1992) Carers Assessment of Satisfaction Index (CASI) and Carers Assessment of Difficulties Index (CADI) were administered, together with Behavioural and Instrumental Stressors in Dementia (BISID) (Keady and Nolan 1996) and Rutter's Malaise Inventory (see Rutter, Graham and Yule 1970; Rutter, Tizard and Whitmore 1970). The interviews lasted between 1 and 4.5 hours with an average time of 2.5 hours. Those interviews with family carers whose relatives had been admitted to care were significantly longer. The methodology for the study, in addition to a discussion on the value of process models in dementia, has been described more fully elsewhere (Nolan *et al.* 1996).

The chapter will now consider the experience of caring for a younger person with dementia using the six-stage model of care as a framework to consider key issues. As highlighted earlier, the model begins with the first stage of 'Building on the past' which, amongst other considerations, explores relationship factors, personality characteristics and belief structures at the (yet to be acknowledged) onset of caregiving. The second stage of 'Recognising the need' is encountered where, particularly in dementia, carers begin to observe subtle changes in the behaviour/cognitions/actions of the person with whom they are concerned, which eventually leads to seeking a formal confirmation of what is happening. This stage is marked by the passages of time and uncertainty. Once a formal confirmation is made, usually in terms of a diagnosis through medical contact, carers enter the decision-making phase involved in 'Taking it on' (Stage 3) before beginning the complexities and dynamics involved in 'Working through it' in Stage 4. At some time, and with a diversity of potential exit points, carers will eventually arrive at the fifth stage of 'Reaching the end' before embarking upon 'A new beginning', which is the sixth and final stage of the model. The threads of each stage, or transition, are held together by a meta concept which we have described as 'maintaining involvement' (for additional discussion see Keady 1997).

Stage 1: Building on the past

As noted earlier, it is essential to recognise that people with dementia and their carers have their own unique biographies and life histories which create a personal experience. However, as the interviews proceeded it became increasingly clear that certain common features emerged which helped better to understand the transition to a caregiving role. These included:

- access to advice, support and information
- the nature, quality and degree of reciprocity in the past relationship
- the nature, quality and degree of reciprocity in the present relationship
- proximity of formal and informal support network
- availability and access to community support
- other related external pressures, such as work demands
- exposure to past experiences of caring
- previous exposure to dementia

- carer belief structures, including marital vows and religious beliefs
- geographical location
- maintenance of individual identity within the relationship
- ability to draw on a range of coping behaviours
- social expectations and perceived pressure from others to carry on caring
- personal ways of managing stress
- gender.

In this sample geographical location was an important factor as the majority of the sample were drawn from a rural population and no specialist services for younger people with dementia were available. However, whilst this undoubtedly complicated the picture, carers often mobilised other types of support and had limited expectations of help.

Central to an understanding of 'Building on the past' is the nature and quality of previous relationships. Identifying these processes gave subtle clues as to the motivating factors involved in continuing to provide care. For instance, one interview with a younger female spouse carer (aged 56) revealed a domestic caregiving relationship which was fraught with difficulties, as this quotation highlights:

> Our relationship has always been bad, no worse than that, dreadful. I mean he was away all the time and even when he came home he acted as if he never wanted to be here. I began to dread him coming home and I only put up with it for the sake of children. They kept us together. You see I got used to leading my own life and since this started [the dementia] he's around the house all the time relying on me for things, like finding out the times of the bus or demanding to know where I've hidden his car keys. Well I just don't want to do anything for him but he is ill, forgetful and that. Everyone would expect me to be there for him but he was never there for me. I feel so trapped and on my own.

As this quote suggests, the past relationship with her husband had been very poor and was having a seriously detrimental effect on their present domestic relationship. Her husband had worked as a long-distance lorry driver even before their marriage some 30 years ago, and whilst initially the carer described their relationship as 'loving and close', this steadily deteriorated with the carer admitting to feeling little or no love for her husband over the last few years of their marriage. It became evident from an early stage in the interview that the carer experienced no pleasure at all in giving care for her husband (a position reinforced by the negative replies to the CASI index) and the conversation was littered with descriptions of the hopelessness of her situation. This undoubtedly influenced the progression and nature of the relationship as the carer continually voiced her desire not to carry on caring, and had taken on the role with no expectation of its success.

For some the meaning attributed to the marital vows of 'for better or for worse' was cited by spouse carers as a reason for entering into, and continuing to deliver, home care. Similarly, holding on to deeply held religious beliefs also shaped the context of care and for this group of carers discontinuing care was not an issue, no matter how problematic the behaviour of the younger person with dementia became.

In situations where there had always been and remained an element of reciprocity in the relationship it was rare for feelings of anger or frustration to be voiced towards the person with dementia. Instead, frustration was either directed toward the carer's own perceived shortcomings – 'I've never had enough patience' – or against the amount of personal and professional support received, particularly in the absence of specialist facilities for the younger person with dementia. Anger was often expressed against the diagnostic procedures and support received from GPs and to support services who provided a service which failed to fit within the carer's own pattern of need. Conversely, it was rare to hear an adult–child carer criticise their own children for failing to provide home care, indeed the reverse was often cited. Responsibility was seen as something to be shared by their own brothers and sisters but not by their children, although as also discussed by Jane Gilliard in Chapter 11, the contribution of teenage children of adult–child carers was either put at a distance, or younger children were immersed in caregiving and encouraged to participate fully, including taking part in intimate tasks such as toileting and dressing. To some extent this position was shaped by domestic living arrangements, but it was also attributable to the belief structures of the adult–child carer.

Stage 2: Recognising the need

Achieving a diagnosis of dementia was, for the carers in this study, a slow, insidious process. Changes in mood, speech and behaviour were viewed with concern by the main supporter, a concern that was initially normalised and discounted. For the carer this was first manifested in a process of noticing (see Wilson 1989a, 1989b) especially in relation to conversation and behavioural changes. For instance, there were subtle changes such as not being able to programme the video, lack of interest in lifelong hobbies, work around the house not being completed to usual standards, an inability to concentrate for long periods, poor telephone skills, withdrawal from social situations and sudden changes in mood. On this latter point, one adult–child carer experiencing the early changes to her father, shared the following observation:

> My Dad started to shout at me for nothing really. He would just get up out of his chair, walk out of the room and slam the door shut. He went upstairs to sit in the bedroom. Mum and I didn't know what was going on as he had never done anything like that before. We thought he was having problems at work so we didn't talk to him about it. But it kept going on.

As intimated by the above experience, 'Recognising the need' is marked by periods of great uncertainty and self-doubt. For some carers this is the most stressful period of the entire caregiving history as they are confronted by behaviours and actions that make very little, if any, sense. It lead to carers facing considerations such as:

- What am I seeing?
- Is this okay?
- This might be serious
- This is serious.

This process could last several months or years and often resulted in a strategy of surveillance where the person exhibiting the (undiagnosed) dementia was carefully watched and their actions screened. With the passage of time, noticing changes in intensity and for the person with (undiagnosed) dementia, as well as the carer, explaining events away satisfactorily became increasingly difficult. This led to carers 'recasting events' to begin to search for other explanations.

Confirming that something serious was wrong was seen as a difficult task and family carers did not automatically tell the person with undiagnosed dementia of their concerns. From the interviews there appeared to be three main ways of managing this process, each being an emotionally painful and cathartic experience:

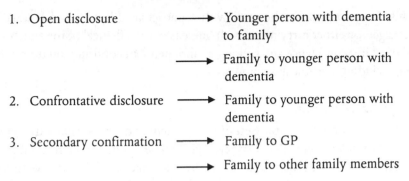

1. Open disclosure   ⟶ Younger person with dementia to family

                           ⟶ Family to younger person with dementia

2. Confrontative disclosure ⟶ Family to younger person with dementia

3. Secondary confirmation   ⟶ Family to GP

                           ⟶ Family to other family members

A brief illustration of each of these points will now be given.

Open disclosure

For family carers and people with dementia this was a time characterised by great uncertainty and emotional release and led to a series of admissions such as:

- 'I've wanted to tell you about this for a long time'
- 'Yes, I am failing'
- 'How long have you known?'
- 'What shall we do now?'

In many ways it was the response to this last statement that determined the outcome of when, and how, to seek professional help. However, a joint decision to seek help together was a relatively rare event within the sample. This mutual process of opening up resulted either in an acceptance of failing abilities and of need for support, or a denial that this was happening. This process of opening up could be initiated either by the younger person with dementia or the family carer.

A process of open disclosure, however, did not always occur. For instance, one of the partners might be ready to disclose their thoughts whilst the other was still recasting events as normal, as one daughter explained:

> I tried to tell my mother about what she was doing and ask her if she recognised it too, but she didn't want to know. I thought I had done all the right things, you know, planned what I was going to say and I waited until there was no one else in the house. She seemed happy enough at first but I couldn't get through to her. She just stopped me stone dead and said there was nothing wrong with her...[pause] but I knew there was.

This situation presents the carer with a particular dilemma and is usually managed by either carrying on with 'increased surveillance' of the situation, or breaking confidence and seeking an independent confirmation from others, including a medical opinion.

Confrontative disclosure

This usually occurred in the heat of the moment and was normally triggered by a particular event. For instance, one female spouse carer remembered screaming at her husband that he 'really was mad' after he had forgotten (again) to turn off the gas taps after heating a tin of beans on the stove. This initial reaction was subsequently followed by a stream of other concerns, a process that was nearly always regretted when the cause of the behaviour became apparent. The impact of such a confrontation was often difficult to evaluate, although a number of carers reported that a confrontative outburst brought no reaction from the person that they cared for, other than silence. It is possible that in this group the person with dementia was able to cope with such an outburst as they had already anticipated such an event, however this is an area that warrants additional investigation.

Secondary confirmation

For some carers the decision to seek medical help was usually described as a breach of confidence towards the cared-for person, as one male spouse carer said: 'she's my wife for God's sake, I didn't want to sound like I was telling tales about her.' However, the decision to seek medical help and guidance was, of itself, an uncertain process. Often the GP might not be the same for both partners and it was consequently difficult for the GP to intervene in such situations. This led to an increasing frustration and uncertainty over the role of the GP in the process as, by this time, carers had accepted that something was seriously wrong and they were looking for confirmation of their beliefs. This is graphically illustrated in the following quotation:

> I went to the doctor because my wife was doing things that I just did not understand. I knew she was ill but nobody would believe me – she couldn't go with me you see and they had to go on what I said. All the doctor said to me was 'Come back again in six months if things have not improved'. Some help that was. (Male carer, aged 54)

Even when arrangements were made to see the person with dementia, reaching a diagnosis of dementia for younger people was not always the first priority. From the sample, depression, the menopause and worry over work were 'diagnoses' that were often reached and offered as an explanation of behaviour. As such the period surrounding diagnosis was an important and traumatic one, and our data suggest that far greater thought should be given as to how information is conveyed at this time. The usual practice was to inform the close family of the suspected diagnosis and leave it to their discretion when, and if, the diagnosis was communicated to the person concerned. This is questionable at the best of times but is particularly so in the case of a younger person who may experience a more rapid progression and loss of competence. Opportunities for younger people with dementia to participate in future decisions which impact upon their lives and that of their families may therefore be denied. There are of course no easy answers to this moral dilemma, but this is an issue that requires an open debate in which the interests of the person with dementia figure prominently.

Stage 3: Taking it on

'Taking it on' is an active, decision-making phase of caregiving which may involve potential sacrifice, such as giving up employment (see Diane Seddon's Chapter 10) and personal time and replacing it with the role of carer. 'Building on the past' is influential in determining whether the decision to take on caregiving is seen as either a positive or uncertain experience. Moreover, there can still be elements of blame towards the younger person with dementia for causing such upheaval, feelings which may accompany the carer throughout the 'long haul' of caring (Rolland 1988).

'Taking it on' raises many questions for service intervention and should be seen as a matter of priority in preparing carers for the potential future(s) that lie ahead. Nolan et al. (1994 – slightly abridged) suggest that informed choice for carers at this time is crucial and that:

- sufficient information on the illness/disease, its progress and treatment should be available for carers to be able to form a realistic picture of the likely future, even if this is only to know that it is uncertain
- on the basis of this information, carers will have a better idea of what is likely to happen; they should also be informed of what they can expect to receive in the way of support and services
- there should be a full exploration of what it is reasonable to achieve in terms of caring; discussion of the fact that there may well be times of emotional turmoil, anger and frustration, and that these are normal

reactions, is useful; furthermore, achievable standards for caring
should be considered – many carers set their own standards too high,
leading to potential disappointment and failure

- the limits and burdens of care should be discussed, as should carers'
  rights to time for themselves; alternatives to home care might also be
  considered, together with what the alternatives are. Setting realistic
  limits can help to ease future decision-making.

Data from our sample would indicate that younger carers were poorly served
at this crucial time with little opportunity to access age-sensitive information
or service options. Indeed, the limitations of statutory service provision for
younger people with dementia (and, of course, for carers) were perceived as a
tremendous hindrance, and only succeeded in adding to the overall weight of
caregiving responsibility as future options were weighed up.

Stage 4: Working through it

The fourth stage of the model is called 'Working through it' and once again
reflects the diversity of the caregiving experience. For example, providing
personal care for a parent was particularly challenging, being described by
one adult male carer as 'going against the natural order of things'. However,
there was also a strong realisation that this was an inevitable part of care and
it was necessary to grit your teeth and get on with it. On the other hand, male
spouse carers continually voiced their concern, and helplessness, at involvement in sanitary care for their wives. During interview, one male carer stated:

> I hate doing that for her. I know it's only once a month but I find it
> embarrassing just buying those things never mind having to find out
> how to use them. I deal with it by bathing her every day until its over. At
> least I know she is clean then and I can put them on [her] the best I can.

During this phase the need for a family-centred, dedicated service for younger people with dementia and their family carers was one of the main themes
to emerge. The backbone of such a service was seen to be day and respite care
together with the provision of local authority community support schemes,
such as home workers. The agency providing such a service was not given
particular importance, the prime consideration being that it was staffed by
people 'who knew what they were doing'. Indeed, the division between the
health and social care sectors often left family carers bewildered and uncertain over who to contact should a need arise.

No one in our sample received a dedicated service of any description. This caused a great deal of distress to family carers, who were both angry and guilty that they had been forced to accept a service intended for older people. Indeed, it was not unusual for the family carer to stop their spouse/parent's attendance at day care centre purely on age-related criteria, in order to protect the younger person with dementia from an adverse experience. The following quotation illustrates this point:

> I couldn't carry on sending him there, it was terrible. I don't want to sound cruel, but everyone at the centre was over 80 and there was my husband, 55, and full of life. He couldn't cope with it and neither could I. I don't think the staff could either, but they never said anything about it to me. They did their best, but in the end I had to take him out of there. I visited him there once and they were all playing bingo, except [my husband] who was beating on the door trying to get out. When he was there I was worried sick all day and never got a moment's rest. At least when he was at home he was with me I could take him out, or he could go to the garage to mess around with his things. (Female carer, aged 54)

The age of onset of dementia also acted to exert a mental pressure on carers who perceived a need to remain in their role, no matter how trapped they felt. Financial worries such as the potential loss of benefits were also a significant factor, as were the limited opportunities for younger people to be admitted into a national health service continuing care facility.

An additional recurring theme from carers who were 'working through it' centred on the need for compensation for financial hardship and loss. The loss of income, coupled with the ineligibility for state or industrial pensions, was a particularly devastating blow for both family carers and younger people with dementia. Fearful of this, at least five spouse carers actively colluded with their partners to maintain an image of normality. All the affected individuals were male and self-employed, and any disruption to their work routine would have had serious financial consequences. Their partners therefore actively reconstructed the daily work patterns of their husbands, covering their slips and working themselves, as one female spouse stated, 'into the ground' to ensure that targets and deliveries were met, and that as little harm as possible came to the family business. Consequently professional services were pushed aside until the couple were both ready to seek help.

Again, there are no easy solutions here, but the availability of some financial compensation would ease the very real fears of family carers and younger

YOUNGER PEOPLE WITH DEMENTIA

people with dementia. However, to achieve this will require a radical shift in public policy, including establishing work-assisted schemes for the younger person with dementia. These could either be located in the normal work environment, or within individually designed sheltered work schemes.

Stage 5: Reaching the end

Carers spoke of gradually being ground down by the weight and responsibility of caring. This was not the result of one factor but a combination of circumstances that led to this outcome, with the absence of satisfactions in providing care being crucial to the decision to contemplate giving up. For some carers, reaching this decision was a relatively easy process and they rationalised that they had done everything possible and that it was time to move on. Such a decision resulted in three processes: first, questioning the care given; second, clarifying alternatives and third, adjusting to the decision. Each of these will now be addressed in turn.

Questioning the care

This strategy was influenced by how the carer had initially approached the caring role. It was not unusual for carers undergoing this process to feel anger towards themselves and frustration towards their inability to carry on. As this son stated during an interview:

> I knew Dad had to go somewhere. I've tried to balance work, family and care for the last six years. I love him but it's time to move on. I wish I could go on but it's come to the end. Someone else will have to do it now.

As this quotation from the study suggests, questioning the care also has a beneficial component with a recognition and awareness that all that could be done had been done. As such, reaching the end and going into care was not always seen as a failure, but also as an achievement that so much had been done to keep the person at home for as long as possible. This realisation leads to a search for help to identify a suitable alternative and included consultation with other family members, and/or discussion with a professional or voluntary agency who has been intimately involved in supporting the carer.

Clarifying alternatives

Once the decision to relinquish care had been made it was vitally important that placement was seen as being the best possible option. However, more often than not, a degree of compromise was required as vacancies and location of the home of choice were not always available, and none exclusively specialised in the care of younger people with dementia. Financial considerations were also important and some carers were shocked to discover that their personal savings would have to be used to pay for care. For some there was considerable personal resentment of this which further influenced the quality of their caregiving relationship, with far more negative perceptions emerging.

Adjusting to the decision

This stage in the process involved a reflection on the past and recent events. There was a need to 'check out' that other people in the family, or friends, also agreed that this placement had been legitimate and in everyone's best interests. This was important to counter the perception that there was also a feeling that other people within a community, or within the family, would see the decision as an indication of failure and of 'giving up' on the situation.

Placement decisions meant placing trust in others and carers stated that this was one of the most difficult periods, as this meant relinquishing control to those outside the immediate relationship. Opening up in this way exposed the younger person with dementia and the family to the outside world, this was often a shock and adjusting to the belief that the person they cared for was, in their words, 'the same as others' brought a range of emotions and coping strategies. Consequently, there was a need to protect themselves from the effects of their decision, with guilt at the decision to institutionalise the cared-for person gradually diminishing over time, leading to an acceptance of the decision. However, this cycle could be resolved quickly or might remain unresolved for several years. Better professional support during this period is critical with other studies suggesting that carers would typically benefit from help in choosing homes and interpreting information on a range of options (Nolan *et al.* 1996).

Stage 6: A new beginning

This final stage of the model considers the carers needs following the forced or voluntary decision to discontinue the caregiving role. The way in which caring was discontinued significantly influenced the way in which carers could resolve issues and move forward. From the study, there would appear to be two dominant stages to this process.

Working through the past

Here the carer strives to find meaning in their caregiving role. It is analogous to the 'recasting of events' function described earlier, but extends to cover the whole process of caregiving, not just discrete events. This is also an active strategy and involves rehearsing events and resolving, and confirming, decisions. Guilt is a feature during this period, a degree of which remained with all younger carers interviewed during this time. Interestingly, dreams about the person with dementia also were in evidence during the interviews. Some were comforting, but others were more psychologically disturbing and hampered the carers' ability to work through the past and commence a new beginning with their life.

Finding new directions

Following institutionalisation or the death of the younger person with dementia, carers expressed the need to find a new direction whilst also preserving their unique contribution to the care of the person with dementia. Finding a new direction was not an easy process. Restructuring family systems following the loss of the person with dementia was extremely stressful. Some younger carers felt that they were at a loose end and that suddenly, after a number of years of caring and investing in the person with dementia, they were no longer useful. Where the younger person with dementia was in institutional care, family carers believed that their lives were on hold and could not progress; this was especially true of the younger carers who felt they were unable to move on as their spouse was still alive. As one 58-year-old spouse stated: 'How long will this carry on? He's been in the hospital for four years now and I want to get on with my life.'

Other carers wanted to leave dementia 'as far behind them as possible' and re-establish networks and interests that existed before the onset of dementia and their transition into care.

Conclusion

Younger people with dementia are presently poorly served in the policy and service arena and much remains to be done to improve the current situation. Certainly, the emergence of dedicated mental health staff, and ideally younger onset dementia multiagency teams, coupled with the provision of specific, age-appropriate assessment and support services represent important first steps.

On the basis of a detailed individual case history written by a spouse carer with the assistance of the authors (Williams *et al.* 1995), it was suggested that the community mental health nurse has a number of 'key roles' to play in providing services to younger carers of people with dementia, including:

- promotion, support and facilitation of new coping skills for family carers

- dynamic assessment of individual, family and community support

- preparation, information and empowerment (PIE) in helping the family carer move forward in their caregiving experiences.

- developing counselling approaches to address carers' feelings of loss and challenge

- adopting the role of 'informed service networker', and liaison with other clinical and voluntary service personnel

- the need to 'be there' for the carer and the younger person with dementia.

The potential implementation of these approaches to carers of younger people with dementia was outlined recently by Keady and Nolan (1997) with effective assessment being linked, in this instance but with generalisable principles, to the nurses' interpersonal skills. This involved the *nurses ability* to *develop*: trust, understanding, empathy, knowledge, listening skills and reliability; and to *provide*: emotional support, practical, financial and legal advice/information, patience, courtesy, sensitive assessment, family and individual interventions, networking, problem-solving techniques and, most important of all, time.

In the absence of age-appropriate and sensitive intervention materials for use with younger people with dementia and their carers, including young children, the development and provision of such resource material would seem a suitable starting place for person-centred and family intervention. This could be implemented via a family model of support based upon identifying and strengthening existing coping patterns, providing age-based information and introducing adaptive cognitive and behavioural problem-solving skills to both younger people with dementia and their family members.

There may also be a need to move assessment and support into the workplace so that younger people with dementia can be afforded the dignity of continuing to work (if they so desire), whilst providing a more sheltered and supervised work environment. However, such work-assisted schemes require financial expenditure which could, perhaps, be met via a personal insurance scheme and/or by central government commitment. Moreover, an emphasis on team working and multi-agency approaches to case identification are crucial if younger people with dementia and their families are to receive a separate and distinct service, including that of individual workers, assessment facilities and residential environments.

With reference to this latter issue, despite an exhaustive search by the authors, little published material specific to the residential assessment facilities of younger people with dementia could be found. There are examples of dedicated residential services for younger people with dementia (see for instance Appendix 2 from *The Care Must be There,* Dementia Relief Trust (1996)), but these remain isolated cases within overall service planning and coordination. This being the case we would see it as both a challenge to, and responsibility of, the nursing profession and other practitioners to tailor existing assessment and screening instrumentation and intervention techniques – such as validation, reminiscence and life review approaches – to fit the needs of younger people with dementia and their families. Adaptations to these indices and approaches would not only advance the cause of dementia care practice in general, but would also highlight the specific needs of younger people with dementia. It is also crucial that health and social care providers strive to influence the policy agenda where younger people with dementia and their families remain on the margins of an already marginalised service.

Finally, it is important that dementia care practitioners develop their roles, identifying new areas of practice so that they can work alongside younger people with dementia and their family carers. It is hoped that the model we have outlined will provide a useful framework in taking work in this area forward.

CHAPTER 13

Designing for the Needs of Younger People with Dementia

Gretta Peachment

Introduction

The first time one sees a trendy 40-year-old in an aged care dementia specific unit and realises the person is not a staff member but a resident, is a shock. Well-dressed, bright eyed as she walked with two staff members, they seemed a group conversing at ease. It was only on joining them one swiftly realised this woman could not initiate conversation nor respond appropriately, that bright looking though she initially appeared, this changed imperceptibly to confusion tinged with panic when she could not contribute beyond a few words. She lived in a house with 12 other people who had dementia and whose average age was 85 years. That she did not see herself as one of them was obvious; it was the staff to whom she cleaved. A new face on the scene, as was the case when the writer arrived to do a review, one was captivated by her welcoming approach which clearly said 'I'm one of you' but which dissipated into confusion when she was unable to sustain the process of a simple greeting.

It became apparent that this lady, Ms R, was one of three younger women with dementia who lived at the residential facility. Mrs D (diagnosed with alcohol dementia) had a high profile. One could not help but be aware of her stress and agitation as she constantly sought for her daughter. Mrs G (diagnosed with vascular dementia) on the other hand was a silent, genial, placid person who strolled around, interfered with no one and was almost invisible in that she impacted so little on the others.

The residential facility had been planned with considerable attention to detail. The L-shaped building had been designed with the lounge/dining areas in one wing, the bedrooms in the other. A doorway at the end of each wing led out to the garden path which arched around the building and led back to the other entrance. Combining both indoor corridor and outside pathway, the two completed a circuit.

The review being undertaken at the time necessitated spending a considerable amount of time in the grounds, charting movement and patterns of behaviour. Staff were taken by surprise at the debriefing of the review to be informed that Mrs D could complete that circuit in under two minutes and that she had done this 27 times in the two-hour review period. This had included 'time out' when she joined anyone who was sitting on a garden bench or in a lounge chair and made her pressing enquiries about her daughter's non-appearance, before jumping up and hurrying on again. Mrs G surprised staff even more, for unnoticed, she had completed the 'circuit' 38 times in the same period.

The lessons from these three observations are not revolutionary but they highlight some of the issues central to the needs of younger people with dementia. The first lady demonstrated the inappropriateness of being housed among aged care residents. She knew she was not one of them and actively sought out people with whom she felt she could identify. Her willingness and eagerness to be part of the staff team highlighted her need for age-appropriate activities. She needed 'work' to do and a role to fulfil. Mrs D and Mrs G illustrate that apart from other manifestations of the disease process the energy levels of young people, demonstrated above in such different ways, are nonetheless different from the older people. Their physical activity needs have to be addressed. In the case of Mrs D, her behavioural pattern, her agility and physical drive made her presence unsettling if not outrightly disruptive to the older, generally more slow-moving clientele. The latter were in fact at risk as she hurriedly turned a corner or brushed past.

These three examples illustrate the need for appropriate housing, grouping, design and care plans for this doubly unfortunate group of people. It is always distressing for all concerned when dementia strips a person of their future and ultimately of their past, but more so when that process is underway at an early age. Misfortune is compounded when due to the smaller number of people affected, systems are not in place to deliver adequate and appropriate care.

The current situation for most of them is that should they require permanent care or even respite care, the only option available is placement in an aged-care facility. Presumably that is going to change in the near future if publications, of which this book is an example, enlighten policy makers on the specific care needs of this vulnerable group. In the meantime one must build on what is already known. Understanding of the designed environment for people with dementia is becoming increasingly sophisticated as different types of needs are identified. Our knowledge of how the environment can support older people with dementia is continually expanding because of the numbers involved. At the same time, other types of dementia and other needs are being investigated. Dementia associated with Huntington's disease presents unique problems. Parkinson's disease, which in the latter stages is not infrequently accompanied by dementia, presents its own brand of design and care challenges (Peachment in press).

There is little documentation on younger onset dementia both clinically and environmentally, and since there is a dearth of operating age-sensitive dementia specific units there are no precedents available to review. This chapter will therefore focus on dementia design per se and question whether or not the principles need to be redefined for the younger clientele. The chapter will also briefly discuss design for Huntington's disease. The often earlier onset of this disease means that they often have similar needs and the manifestation of their dementia, which is primarily of frontal lobe involvement, presents some commonalities, at certain levels, between the two groups.

Dementia design

Many of the needs of people with dementia do not differ fundamentally from the rest of the community. Those things which give each and every one of us comfort, security, pleasure and sensory satisfaction are constants despite the disease process. As cognitive deficits mount, the built environment needs to assist in a number of ways. Due to the nature of the disease, the longer term memory outlasts the more immediate, the place that many are seeking therefore is in the past. 'Home' no longer exists, either socially or physically. It helps if the present dwelling, if it is a permanent care facility, has an ambience where the transition from past to present is not jarring. This is important also as the disease progresses, for place and presentation can cue people to respond more appropriately when there is confusion of their role and how to function within the environment.

A modern example is the airport lounge with its vast spaces, where seating is designed for transitory use and there is a complete lack of personal statement. The airport lounge tells you to move on. Sadly this is not totally dissimilar to the message given out in some large permanent care institutions where the 'lounge' is a sparse hall-like room with inappropriate seating around the perimeter. Such a room not infrequently doubles as lounge, activity or therapy room, and not surprisingly confusion is increased under these circumstances.

In contrast, a smaller lounge room, carpeted if culturally and climatically appropriate, with soft lighting, drapes, comfortable seating, a fireplace, pictures and mementos, encourages appropriate behaviour. Good design for the younger group with dementia is no different in this respect. Change will be in appropriate soft furnishings, not in room size or role. The long-term memory of a 50–60-year-old would be 40–50 years ago, spanning World War II and postwar years. This makes an interesting challenge. Design responding to the social upheavals of those times in a most distinctive way and individual assessments would be needed to identify the dominating memories of that period, for both social and environmental recall.

Grouping

Most people did not grow up with 30 or so others in the same house. Care situations, if they have to house such numbers, need to be arranged so that small groups can live together and scale does not increase tension and confusion. When the opportunity to build presents itself, a cluster of houses set within secure grounds is the model most favourably viewed today. This creates the opportunity to maintain a domestic scale, particularly if one has the luxury of designing houses for small numbers. Eight people together is a group large enough for social interaction and small enough for bonding of staff and families. Economic realities however, in the form of financially viable staffing levels for 24-hour care, mean that permanent care facilities today, in Australia at least, have to be artfully arranged so that 15 together look, and hopefully feel, like two subgroups of seven or eight.

Physical status

This number may present problems for the younger onset group. Their often higher level of physical fitness means that their energy levels also need to be considered. Fifteen people may be unmanageable and their range of needs too diverse. Aggressive behaviour has always been an aspect of dementia and has an impact far beyond the numbers involved. When manifest in a younger, fitter person this problem may be of different proportions. The average age of those in permanent care is 85 years old, the average number of diagnoses per person on admission appears to be about eight. People with younger onset dementia are likely to present a very different picture. Dementia may be their only diagnosis. Some differences can be anticipated; for example though they may have perceptual problems as part of the disease process this is less likely to be compounded by vision impairments such as age-related maculopathy which reduces central vision so that a person can only see around the peripheries. This condition, like that of cataracts, is associated more with ageing. Sexual expression may be more evident among younger people, and may or may not be combined with disinhibition. The availability of privacy, both for the individual and when partners, family members and children visit, will have consequences for design aspects.

Design: a sensory approach

As with dementia within any age group, an environment which puts emphasis on sensory awareness is one which is investing in peoples' strengths rather than one which relies on diminishing cognitive skills. While the latter declines, the senses remain largely intact for a much longer period. Sensory knowledge has always been recognised, but is a tool which has been largely overlooked in dementia care, where the need to address behavioural problems seems to dominate the initial agenda. It is through our senses however that we relate to space, to shape and depth, to time, to movement, to light, to touch, to the quality and structure of everything around us, to reality. As one of the aims of dementia care is to keep that connection with 'reality' as viable as possible, for as long as possible, sensory stimulation or enhancement is a tool to be exploited.

This chapter includes a case study on 'The Village', a dementia-specific unit commissioned in 1994. An interest in sensory assessment arose through some anomalies observed in the post-occupancy evaluation of that facility where it was found that cognitive testing did not necessarily correlate with sensory awareness of the environment. On admission each person had undergone a daily routine of 45 minutes of orientation. This was to inform the person about which house they lived in, which room within the house was theirs and which colour would assist them. Evaluation later showed that some of those with higher Mini-Mental State (Folstein, Folstein and McHugh 1975) and Dementia Hierarchic Scale scores did not necessarily find their house and room as well as some whose score was as low as 3/30. Even taking into account that the disease is degenerative and that a person's situation could have deteriorated in the intervening six months, it begs the question how far does sensory awareness of the environment compensate for cognitive decline? This is an area inviting research for the future. For the present however, and with these findings in mind, design will be discussed throughout this chapter from a sensory perspective. Of the five sensory modalities vision, smell, taste, touch and sound, movement could probably be added to this list, but vision remains our dominating sense. Vision combined with another modality is even more effective.

Visual access

Reference has already been made to the need for rooms to cue people for appropriate behaviour. Confusion about where one is, where one is going and how one gets there, needs to be recognised by planners. Buildings need to offer features which reduce the stress and agitation that accompanies these aspects of the disease. Buildings designed for full visual access assist in this manner. The toilet on view from the bedroom assists continence. The example given is that if a person with dementia wakens with a full bladder, they may not recognise the messages being sent to the brain, but if the cueing is there, i.e. the toilet is on view, they may go onto 'automatic pilot' and respond appropriately.

On leaving the bedroom it is helpful if the person is not confronted with a number of decisions. If left or right both appear to lead nowhere, such as a dead end or a bend in the corridor which masks the path to the kitchen, confusion is increased. Full visual access means decision making is simplified, the number of alternatives is reduced and the visual cueing therefore enhanced.

Cueing

A range of ideas have been used to assist people to locate their own bedroom door. Strong colours, tactile features, reminiscence in the form of the person's long-term memory of the front door associated with their childhood, memory boxes containing significant items, all require individual assessment to locate the key for each individual. The most effective tool is to assess who can still recognise their own name. A simple name plate remains the most effective measure. A down light which illuminates the nameplate may increase effectiveness.

Light itself is an effective cueing device. For example, it is estimated that the amount of light required by a 75-year-old is almost three times that of a 20-year-old. The need for strong lighting is compromised however if it produces glare. Glare from reflected light on shiny floor surfaces strongly affects people with vision deficits. It is one of the issues which influences the decision to use carpet in dementia care units, this is despite the fact that incontinence can be a problem. High lumen levels and glare will not be as problematical for younger people with dementia because of the age differences and general health standards. 'Smart houses' in Norway link technology with lighting for cueing behaviour and to help prevent falls. During the hours of darkness, as a person rises from the bed, the light in the appropriately positioned toilet comes on. The bedroom light also comes on but begins dimly and gradually increases to full strength. (Bjømeby in press).

Sound

Elevated noise levels are related to increased confusion, agitation and aggression. Dramatic changes have been noted by staff who have accompanied people throughout the transition from ward situations with vinyl floors and 'hard' surfaces to the small, noise-reducing environments of a domestic scale cluster house. Impaired thought processing, decision making and attentiveness are compounded when there is overstimulation, of which noise is a prime contributor. Noise reduction, combined with the less hurried movement of carers, create an enabling environment for people with dementia. This is not to say that people with dementia do not like to make a noise themselves and it is envisaged that this may be particularly the case with a younger clientele, as it is with a number who have Huntington's disease, but there is a difference between a stimulating environment and one which suffers from overstimulation.

Taste and smell

Furthering our investigations into sensory responses a colleague and myself were recently dismayed at the poor response of people with dementia to smell and taste. With or without visual cues few could identify many items in either category. Gustatory tests were based on sweet, sour, bitter and salt and a variety of tastes were offered. The responses were only put into context when staff members underwent the same test. The results were not dissimilar. This suggests that if people cannot see what they are eating their responses are depressed. This has major implications regarding food presentation, particularly when pureed or vitamised food, is served. For younger clients it is even more important to provide attractive presentations where taste is assisted by visual cues such as colour, shape, form and texture and enhanced by the smell of food being prepared need to be incorporated to create a robust environment. This is important not only to maintain appetite and body weight, but to address quality of life issues.

Touch

Tactile responses demand attention for the skin is the largest sensory organ of all. A variety of tactile surfaces and textures are needed to stimulate a person's response to the world around them. The wind, the sun, rain, the sea, running water, sand are all necessary external stimuli. Within a house a variety of experiences should be available: varying surfaces, seating, upholstery, cutlery, and wall hangings increase tactile experiences. How one likes to be touched on the other hand, could almost be classified as internal stimuli.

Case study 1: 'The Village'

(A 44 bed unit in Perth, Western Australia)

To illustrate the practical application of much that has been referred to above, the following case study looks at a dementia-specific unit commissioned in 1994. Designed for 'at risk' people who require a secure environment it was not done with younger onset people in mind but in the intervening years three younger people have now taken up residence.

The case study may stimulate debate as to the pros and cons of integrating 'younger' with 'older' people as well as identifying suggested points of effective design.

The site utilised for this project was a corner block. Five houses were designed to face a two-street frontage. The houses were angled so that small connecting walkways not only formed a secure parameter but enabled staff to move from house to house with ease at night. A clubhouse completed the built environment and this was located within the park-like grounds established at the back of the houses (see Figure 13.1).

Although designed to house either eight or ten people, the aim had been to achieve a domestic feel. The style of all the houses was 'Federation'. This fitted in with the street-scape and is a style which, although not contemporary, is still popular today. Younger people would still seek to buy existing houses in older suburbs from such stock, or use the design motifs in new houses. To differentiate the houses, different coloured bricks were used.

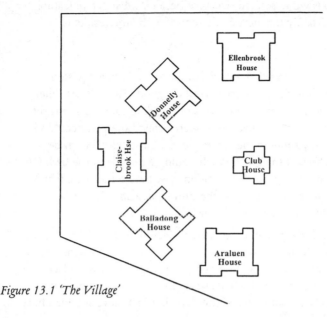

Figure 13.1 'The Village'

Once a resident, life revolved around each 'home' house, the grounds and the clubhouse. As the grounds were open at the rear, residents could also 'visit' any other of the houses. The back view of the house for the people who lived there was therefore of high priority, and as it presented as a street-scape, confused residents would need some strategies in place to assist them locate their house.

External cueing strategies

- *Name plate.* Each house had a traditional name plate mounted on the wall.

- *Wall plaque.* A large, decorative wall plaque was also mounted on the wall. Each plaque had a simple motif, a fish, a bird, a flower, a fruit (a bunch of grapes), a sun figure. The motifs were boldly expressed in primary colours. To reinforce the cue, a transparency to match the motif was on the glass door so that as a person left the house and went into the garden they were reminded of 'their' symbol.

- *Garden furniture.* On the veranda each house had a setting of garden furniture. These five distinct types each had a different shape and colour. The central house had a large rose arbour and this white painted structure became a distinctive feature and certainly the most easily identified by the residents.

Internal cueing strategies

- *Total visual access*: To reduce confusion and assist decision making the design concentrated on good visual access. There were no corridors so the stress of deciding to go left or right was removed. The bedrooms were around the perimeter and the family room in the central space. En suites off each bedroom housed the toilet which could be seen from the bed. On leaving the bedroom the resident saw before them the family room which incorporated the dining area and the kitchen, both of which were totally visible.

- *Colour*: Strong colour was used to identify each bedroom door. Cueing devices were necessary as so many doors opened onto the family room. Moulding of differing patterns was placed on each door to assist both visual and tactile recognition. The bedroom colour matched the door but in a more subdued hue.

- *Name plates*: All residents were assessed for reading skills and those who could still recognise their name were given name plates.

- *Bedspreads*: Unless the family supplied their own bedspread, the original coloured one from our own stock was to be used consistently by staff.

Furniture

Furniture that was ageless was chosen, where possible, to assist the bridging of the present and the past. This necessitated buying some pieces from auction rooms and second-hand stores. New furniture was designed with certain outcomes in mind. Dining tables were wooden based with rounded wooden edging while the insert was in a contrasting colour. Again this was colour coded from house to house, but the colours were also chosen to assist those with visual impairment and those with figure ground problems (difficulties in identifying an object against its background.) Deficits in this area are common to many people with dementia. Coping with white porridge in a white bowl, identifying sugar and milk in white containers and all on a white tablecloth is a recipe for disaster for many. Figure ground and depth perception deficits are helped by some form of contrast.

- *Seating*: Seating is a subject all of its own. Earlier investigations had shown the need for well-thought-out and well-designed furniture. This assists greatly in the care for those with dementia (Wagland and Peachment 1996). Within each house five different types of seating were offered to the resident, in the lounge room, family room, bedroom, dining room and outdoors. Each group were not only of a different shape and offering different forms of comfort, but each was to offer a different visual and tactile experience. Linen, cotton, suede, tapestry, velvet, jacquards and wood all have a distinctive feel. This was used as well as shape and pattern for sensory stimulation, to help identify a favoured chair, and to give each house a separate identity. Two-seater settees were used as well as single chairs. This cued for behavioural patterns of social interaction within the group. It also offered families the opportunity to sit close to each other when visiting: husband and wife, mother and daughter.

Pictures and artefacts

Pictures were chosen which made a clear statement. Clear colours, simple themes, pictures with a narrative element, animals and fruit were all considered suitable. Impressionist paintings and abstract paintings were avoided. The busy lines and blurring of colours appeared disturbing to those who were already confused. Artefacts were chosen to not only be admired, but also to be handled.

Lighting

Lighting proved problematical with such a large family room in the centre of each house. Despite assurances from the architects that four skylights would be sufficient, this has proved not to be the case. Inadvertently however, it works well as a cueing device to encourage people to go into the garden. The main source of natural light is from the double glass doors leading from the family room to the outside. This appears to entice people to venture out and we have the type of climate where this is possible for a large part of the year.

Garden

- *Design aspects*: The garden is large and park-like in its dimensions. It has been designed foremost with people who 'wander' in mind. The pathways are not straight but meander and wind their way through the grounds and taking the fastest route is prevented by the lack of symmetry. In the early growth stages of the garden, the low plants appeared not to be seen and were trampled underfoot by those with figure ground problems. As the plants have grown, the design philosophy appears to be working increasingly well.

- *Horticultural aspects*: The garden was designed with colour, contrast, variety, smell, taste, shade, sound and reminiscence in mind. The seasons were emphasised by planting deciduous trees (Australian trees are largely non-deciduous). Each house garden outside the rear door was colour coded, for example, the first house had a yellow theme, the second blue, then red, white and pink.

- *Social aspects*: Within the garden was a workshop for anyone who wished to potter. An outdoor barbecue was available for social events such as family gatherings. A car, permanently parked in the grounds, gave opportunities for activity. People could wash and polish the car and often people just liked to sit in it.

The clubhouse

Set in the heart of the grounds was the clubhouse. A lounge room was designed for a certain purpose and its size, proportions and furnishings were suitably cued for certain activities. The clubhouse was furnished in a manner which aimed to give a different message. The patterned carpet was chosen for its 'game' theme, and encircled a small dance floor in the centre. The seating suggested that one could stay for a while, but that it was not a lounge room. The building in its size and with its vaulted ceiling suggested community gatherings.

Being escorted and supervised when participating in events with the wider community often makes inroads on staff time which is not always sustainable or available at the right time. A clubhouse, set within secure grounds, offers much scope and a stand-alone building has many advantages. Such advantages are listed below:

- going to the clubhouse is an outing – one has to put on a coat, take an umbrella, dress appropriately for the weather

- it is an outing away from 'home'

- activities in the clubhouse can take on the role of 'work': after breakfast one has a job to do, to go to the clubhouse; after the morning activities the 'job' is to go home for lunch. This can be repeated in the afternoon
- although group as well as one-to-one activities can take place within the houses, group activities offering increased opportunities for socialisation are easily managed within a clubhouse setting; such activities as the gardening club, Tai Chi and musical events offer participation in a variety of ways
- clubhouses offer the increased opportunity to involve families and the community. Once a week the clubhouse becomes a restaurant with tables appropriately dressed where permanent residents and their visitors can dine together. Evening dances, church services, birthday and anniversary celebrations bring families together in an environment which offers more scope for either privacy or socialisation.

The case study offers a design model which specifically addresses a number of problems associated with caring for people with dementia in a permanent care setting. Some of these principles are:

- group small numbers of people together
- create an ambience to which they can relate
- design for sensory stimulation
- design to assist decision making and reduce stress
- single bedrooms with en suites
- good internal visual access
- cue for wayfinding
- cue for function
- design for social interaction
- appropriate seating
- well-designed outdoor areas.

These principles can be used not just for permanent care, but for respite care and for domestic and supported housing. The same principles can be used and adapted to be age-sensitive for younger people with dementia. With minor modifications such as curtaining, chair shape and choice of upholstery fabrics, furniture selection, modern light fixtures, appropriate reminiscence material, artefacts and pictures, 'The Village' might offer a functional and appropriately stimulating facility for some younger people, if remaining within ordinary housing or other supported housing is no longer a viable option.

Multisensory centres

An additional aspect of design and care not included in the case study and one which has been a more recent development is the inclusion of a Snoezelen, or multisensory room and programme. Developed originally for children with learning disabilities (Hulsegge and Verheul 1987) it was discovered to be very beneficial when used as a therapy for older people with dementia. It holds great potential to be developed for younger people with dementia. While in its original form, Snoezelen was an interactive, recreational activity seen to be failure free for participants, in its adaptation for older people with dementia a more passive form has been found to be most beneficial. Measurement of results is proving to be difficult, despite the fact that practitioners give anecdotal accounts of dramatic, short-term changes in behaviour. Speech and communication appear to be significantly improved, though temporarily, while aggression is also reported to be tempered. A more consistent report is that people are more alert and take a more sharpened interest in their surroundings following a Snoezelen session.

Individual sensory assessments are required before entering such a programme and this in itself assists all forms of individual care planning, not just the Snoezelen programme. The amount of information gleaned from multisensory assessment helps identify, irrespective of cognitive state, where a person 'is' today. Understanding a person's sensory response enables a carer to share this experience and this can form a vital non-verbal communication. Many activities are first concentrated in a 'white room'. Extraneous stimulation is removed and focused stimulation based on prior assessment is introduced with specific outcomes in mind. With any one or a combination of, for example, bubble tubes, mirrors, oscillating lights, mood wheels, appropriate music (which is often New Age as this is related to body rhythms), a very relaxing, almost hypnotic effect is achieved. Tactile stimulation, how a person likes to be touched and where, such as with a neck or a foot massage can be added. Aromatic oils offer olfactory stimulation.

Alongside the material aspects of multisensory centres in dementia care is a philosophy which is based on careful assessment, both before and after the session, a shared experience between the person with dementia and the carer and the establishment of trust and confidence between these two people. As such, it is an eminently suitable tool for use in the care of people with dementia and offers particular potential both in the passive form described above and, perhaps, a more robust recreational and interactive form suitable for younger more physically active people.

The environment for people with Huntington's disease

The particular needs of people with Huntington's disease have been described in Chapter 6. Design needs to address, where possible, the results of frontal lobe deterioration of the brain which are often manifest in distinctive patterns of behaviour and, equally, motor deficits, which result in distinctive physical impairments. Designing for this range of needs is a challenge. The residential facility often needs to be a 'safe harbour'. Design is particularly challenged under these circumstances to marry together 'home' and 'function'.

Social environment

People with this condition need an environment which offers personal space, privacy, dignity, stability, continuity, care, consideration and comfort. This does not mean a palliative care approach. Rather, the driving philosophy of care is to strive to maintain independence through a concentrated physiotherapy programme, to capitalise on strengths with occupational therapy and nursing support, to create opportunities and to offer challenges that contribute to a quality of life.

Buildings therefore need to be domestic in scale, allowing for small groups to live together as an extended family. Offering alternative spaces is very important to this group. Single bedrooms allow for the privacy people need and adjoining rooms can answer for those who wish to share. Due to the diverse behavioural manifestations of the disease social dynamics can be addressed more effectively if options are available. Within the home there is the personal and private sphere, the single bedroom. Shared space among a small group is available in the lounge and dining rooms. A clubhouse or amenities area on site widens the options for communal activities with extended families in an atmosphere of tolerance and understanding.

Physical environment

As with people with Parkinson's disease and for the same reasons, (i.e. impaired thought processing in planning and sequencing), design should be simple. All areas should be spacious, since gait instability and jerking movements may need to be accommodated. The extra space is also required to allow people who, apart from the physical difficulties described, also have perceptual deficits. Rounded edges, padded sharp corners, countersunk handles where appropriate, are recommended. Sliding doors are easier for those with involuntary movement if the door handle is a long moulded form that is attached from top to bottom. No matter where people connect with it they can effect movement.

Communication

Any discussion on this subject begins with reference to good seating techniques. Poor posture combined with muscle rigidity leads to decreased lung function. The reduced capacity and control of respiration affects the quality of the voice. Impaired vocal strength leads to uncoordinated speech sounds. The first requirement of communication is to have the person positioned in appropriate, individualised seating. In the earlier stages a high, winged-back, comfortable armchair which fits snugly around a person and gives good support offers comfort and security while reducing visual and auditory distractions from the back and sides. A mini environment can thus be created to aid direct communication face to face.

Offering security, comfort and reducing distractions is necessary, not just to assist cognitive functions, but because of the person's short attention span. Noise, activity and overstimulation are not appropriate – the environment needs to be supportive by being restful. Noise-absorbent floor coverings such as carpet reduce noise levels substantially. Wall hangings, though not so effective, still contribute.

Meal times

People with Huntington's disease burn calories at a very high rate for several reasons. They need food not just to replace this rapid burnout but because if one can keep up the body weight symptoms are more controllable. Lose weight and the symptoms are often exacerbated. 'Food is medicine' is a doctrine in some facilities for this group of people. The aim is to maintain body weight plus 10 per cent. There are, however, many problems associated with the swallowing symptoms of people with Huntington's disease. Three major ones are mentioned here. First, at times they eat too fast; they are hungry and have instant gratification needs; second, due to poor breath control there are sudden unexpected gasps for air; and third there is swallow/respiration uncoordination. Together these problems may cause coughing and choking.

Seating, emphasised so much in this chapter, is again a fundamental aspect of care. A meal is a social event and people respond to this depending on their personality traits. Seating which offers comfort and postural support is required by all at any stage. While still physically independent, chairs should be light enough to move about so a person can sit up to the table and move away without staff intervention if they have the ability to do so. Correct upright posturing to assist swallowing and decrease the risk of aspirating can sometimes be a matter of life or death. In advanced stages there is a need for a quiet environment so that concentration on swallowing can be assisted.

A circular table on a heavy pedestal base, operated with a gas lift, means the table can be raised and lowered to accommodate wheelchairs. Colour contrasts on the table assist those with visual deficits. The dining room should be as visually welcoming, as the smells are enticing.

Food preparation when the diet is soft or pureed has always been a challenge. The compartmentalised plate with scoops of vitamised food is not only a thoroughly unappetising prospect due to its blandness, consistency and presentation, but also has childish connotations. The concept of serving moulded or shaped foods has been round for a little while. Through the use of thickeners and moulds, pulverised foods can be reshaped to demonstrate the original form, for example, pork chops, fish, chicken shapes and fruit. It cues people by informing them what they are eating and encourages appetite and appropriate responses. Chefs should be encouraged to be innovative in their presentation and to identify new products as they come on the market.

The built environment, the sensory environment and the care plan

The design aspects discussed up to this point are basic steps in the care of people with a specific type of neurodisability. A therapeutic environment should be a holistic concept where the built environment, the sensory environment and the care plan contribute to each other.

The following case study is an example of this approach. (Names have been changed to preserve anonymity.)

Case study 2: Peter

Peter, 48 years, is married with a son and daughter. He worked as a crane driver, was diagnosed with Huntington's disease in 1991 and has been recently admitted to permanent care. His current situation is as follows.

Insight

Peter has retained his insight. He is both distressed at knowing the future and seeing it in the people around him as well as being relieved that he is with 'the family', the small coterie of people he has associated with at the Huntington's Association. He needs to both mix with and withdraw from the group. Creating a private space for him is important.

Noise

Peter is distressed by loud noises. He needs to be housed away from the noise hub of the facility. When he is with the group and noisy activities are in progress, he needs to be offered alternatives as he is unmotivated and may not remove himself of his own volition until his behaviour indicates distress.

He enjoys watching football on TV and videos played in a quieter area may well suffice at these times. Alternatively, if he is distressed and as we know can no longer go to concerts, CDs and videos may be made available. These are appropriate gifts for his family to consider. He is very family-orientated and gets distressed by their inability to stay throughout the day. One son lives over 1000 kilometres away and has a small child. A video of family updates may relieve his distress when he needs his time alone.

Communication

Peter has some slurring of speech but can easily make himself understood. At present he has three abilities which should be harnessed:

- he can make himself understood verbally
- he can read short passages
- although he answers questions spontaneously, delayed recall allows him to correct himself if the answers are incorrect.

Now is the time to record his voice for use later in conjunction with a communication panel if this seems appropriate. This is not only creating a tool for the future but will be important to Peter who is striving to maintain his individuality in a group setting. Other communication systems can be introduced while he can respond to written instructions.

Peter's ability to read short passages can be put to other uses. He expresses a love of nature and of gardens. Magazines with vivid pictures and accompanying text may be useful for someone like Peter and should be readily available. His short attention span means longer passages in books will not be successful.

Olfactory

Peter could not identify many smells but when shown plants he could name a number of them. Access to a garden would give him solace and also answer his need to get away from others. Raised garden beds are not always available but a terracotta trough placed at bench height is an alternative. After tending it can be placed outside his bedroom door or window; this states ownership. Mints, fragrant geraniums, curry plants are easy care and aromatic, while others can be grown for their colour and beauty.

Colour

Peter's preference for reds and greens could be incorporated into a gardening programme. Colour can be used as a personal statement within his own personal space. A picture set in a red mounting, a green bedspread are little touches which could further demonstrate his individuality.

Tactile

Peter dislikes physical expressions of affection unless they come from his family. In terms of body language, it is no surprise that he prefers a back massage to any other form. It lessens the intimacy of the procedure and precludes eye contact. The use of oils during this therapy could be linked to his garden and nature interests. Citrus oils and fragrances, soothing and beneficial to his skin yet evocative of the garden, create a vehicle for conversations that are non-threatening and can be related to happier times in the past, particularly family events when he lived in the country.

Conclusion

Design for dementia is a specialised area, yet at the same time many aspects of design have universal appeal because they arise from basic human needs. As such, dementia design can be, and should be, the basic design model for all care situations. Design to cope with functional disabilities which accompany other disease symptoms can be superimposed on this model. The complexity of the requirements of people with, for example, Huntington's disease should not cloud the fact that good dementia design with informed modifications will also serve those purposes well.

Design for younger people with dementia needs to be addressed. Poor design increases the problems people must cope with, it contributes to depression, increases family and staff stress and creates time-consuming situations. Design will never supplant care, but good design which is sensory enhancing and respects individual preferences can become a therapeutic agent to assist and contribute to best practice and to the quality of life for those who require our care.

Further reading

Iwasaki, K. and Holm, N.B. (1989) 'Sensory treatment for the reduction of stereotypic behaviour in persons with severe multiple disabilities.' *Occupational Journal of Research 9*, 170–183.

Moffat, N. *et al.*(1993) *Snoezelen: An Experience for People with Dementia.* Derbyshire: Rompa.

Morris, M. (1995) 'Dementia and cognitive changes in Huntington's disease. Behavioral neurology of movement disorders.' In W.J. Weiner and A.E. Lang (eds) *Advances in Neurology, Vol. 65.* New York: Raven Press.

Zolton, B. (1996) *Vision, Perception and Cognition: A Manual for the Evaluation and Treatment of the Neurologically Impaired Adult,* 3rd edn.

PART FOUR

Practice Developments

CHAPTER 14

Younger People with Dementia
Psychosocial Interventions
Bob Woods

Introduction

This chapter addresses the key question of what can be done to assist younger people with dementia and their supporters. Greater awareness of the prevalence of dementia in younger people and of its impact must be followed by efforts to develop and implement interventions of real value to those affected. Identification and assessment which do not lead on to useful systems of therapy, support and care will be of limited value.

Most attention is usually given to the new drugs which are now becoming available, and for which great hopes exist. This is an area of rapid progress (and, it should be said, considerable media hype). The first group of drugs to be licensed for use in Alzheimer's disease operate on the chemical pathway in the brain most closely involved in memory function – the cholinergic neurotransmitter system. Tacrine (available in the USA) and donzepil hydrochloride (Aricept) fall into this category. Others will undoubtedly follow in their wake, with some targeted at vascular dementia. Here already aspirin is widely viewed as a useful means of slowing down decline through it's role in preventing further mini-strokes. At least for the foreseeable future, it seems likely that the medications which become available will, at best, slow down the rate of decline in function in the person with dementia, and in so doing will ameliorate the difficulties of the situation experienced in a proportion of cases. 'Cures' are not yet realistically on the agenda as far as dementia is concerned. It is important to bear in mind the diversity of types of dementia encountered with younger people – each will require it's own tailored pharmacological approach. Even with what we now consider to be

246 YOUNGER PEOPLE WITH DEMENTIA

Alzheimer's disease, it is likely that distinct subtypes will eventually be identified, which in turn may respond differently to drug treatments. In relation to the drugs acting on the cholinergic system, it is well established that a number of other neurotransmitter pathways are also malfunctioning, particularly in younger people with Alzheimer's disease. The current drugs can then only be a partial approach to treatment, tackling only one part of the overall picture.

In this chapter the emphasis will be on psychosocial approaches to intervention, which are likely to be needed whatever welcome pharmacological breakthroughs are around the corner. The pattern or rate of progression may be altered and there may well be a need for improved assessment and diagnosis of the type of dementia present, as drugs with more specific action are developed, but dementia will still be with us, changing lives and presenting unforeseen challenges.

Much has been written concerning psychosocial interventions with people with dementia (e.g. Miesen and Jones 1997; Woods 1996). The emphasis has tended to be on older people with dementia, presumably because younger people with a dementia are in the minority, and because many services for dementia have developed from and within services for older people. Most of the work that has been carried out with older people has direct relevance for younger people and their families. Best practice will in any case emphasise the importance of an individual, tailored approach; the range of diversity amongst older people with dementia in fact would probably be as great as any age differences in needs of people with dementia. It should not therefore be any different in principle to produce an individualised intervention for a 35-year-old person with dementia as opposed to one for an 85-year-old. However, there are some aspects that do need careful consideration, and may have a particular bearing on the situation of the younger person with dementia.

1. The rate of progression in the underlying disorder may generally be greater in younger people with dementia. There will still be considerable variation, of course, but there will be a particular need for responses to be timely and flexible.

2. The social context of the disorder will be different from that encountered with most older people. For many, the disorder will be impinging, initially at least, on the person's work. It may well be here that the first difficulties are evident. If and when the person can no longer work, the loss of the work role, and of the financial rewards associated with it, may

affect the person's self-esteem as well as leading to potential financial problems. The younger person is also more likely to have responsibility for childcare and/or to have dependent children. Again, if and when the dementia makes it difficult to fulfil these roles, the person's self-image may well be damaged. The involvement of young children brings into the picture issues regarding the well being and protection of the interests of the children. In contrast, for most older people developing dementia the transition into retirement has already occurred, and any childcare responsibilities are likely to be once-removed as a grandparent, perhaps. Although many older people do have significant social roles, there is a tendency for them to occupy a less pivotal position than previously. Perhaps all concerned recognise the eventual inevitability of mortality, and accordingly less is expected of older people in these roles.

3. There is a sense in which loss of memory – alongside other losses of strength, vigour and power – is almost an expectation of later life in our society, to the extent that a person in advanced old age who retains memory and intellectual power or physical fitness becomes noteworthy almost as an exception to the general 'rule'. Memory loss can then acceptably be attributed to age by many who develop a dementia in later life. If confronted with an evident memory lapse it can always be 'explained' as a sign of ageing, without having to enter into a realisation of a more profound loss of function. In this way, for the older person dementia is 'timely' in that it occurs in the phase of life when such difficulties are to be expected. Generally in developmental studies the timeliness of an event is related to the relative ease of adaptation to its impact. For example, an older person adjusts more readily to the death of a spouse than to the death of an adult child, which has occurred outside of the time of the lifecycle when death is, if not predictable, at least not unexpected. Although great pains have been taken in recent years by researchers and professionals working in the field to stress that dementia is not part of the normal ageing process, the public perception remains, fuelled by the exponential increase in the prevalence with age. For younger people with dementia, attributions of the cause other than age will be prominent. For Creutzfeldt-Jakob disease (CJD), there is a possible external cause through the link with Bovine Spongiform Encephalopathy (BSE). For other types of dementia, some family members will find ways of blaming themselves or will find another external event that seemed to trigger the sequence of events. To seek a reason for suffering is a very common response; often reasons are not easily found, and

those who might be providing mutual support and comfort enter into cycles of blame, recrimination and guilt, which tend to be destructive for all concerned. We must add to this already potent mix the greater likelihood in younger people with dementia that a genetic mechanism of transmission may be at work, with ensuing guilt feelings in the aware person with dementia and fear for the future in children and close blood-relatives. Each person's family situation will of course be unique; each will have their own way of coping and of seeking to understand. What younger people with dementia and their families cannot do is to hold on to the age-attribution as an early source of support while a more sophisticated understanding develops.

4. Typically, the older person will have a number of physical health problems, often chronic in nature, on which the dementia is superimposed. Many physical health and sensory changes become more common with advancing age, and an important component of dementia assessment in the older person is to carry out a full physical health evaluation. Often, the person's mental state is worsened by sensory loss, physical health problems or the combination of medications being taken to assist with these. The younger person, on the other hand, is less likely to have other major illnesses (although a full evaluation of physical health is no less essential), and generally initially will be fitter and stronger than the average older person. This situation has advantages, of course, in that the person will require less medical input and will be able potentially to participate in a broader range of physical activities. However, in the context of challenging behaviour, in situations where the person feels frustrated, where communication breaks down or where the person loses control, potentially the strength of the outburst may be much more difficult to contain within safe limits.

5. Working with younger people with dementia may raise particular issues for professional helpers. With older people with dementia, the professional helper is inevitably younger and although he/she may identify with a younger carer, will be unlikely to identify so closely with the person with dementia. With a younger person with dementia, the helper will perhaps have much more directly in common, and will need to be aware of the risks of overidentification, of projecting his/her own reactions, fears and anxieties on to the person with dementia, at the cost of the sensitive, in-depth listening that is required to discern the person's own feelings and reactions. Clinical supervision has an important part to

play in assisting helpers to identify the impact of their own feelings or their relationship with the person with dementia and other supporters.

Interventions with the person with dementia

General principles

1. THE PRIMACY OF VALUES

Although it has long been recognised that the attitudes and values underlying the care provided have a critical influence on the person with dementia (e.g. King's Fund 1986), the work of Kitwood has brought this into sharp focus over the past few years (e.g. Kitwood 1997). Kitwood argues that the social environment surrounding the person with dementia has the power to increase the person's apparent level of disability and even to accelerate the rate of decline. The features of the social environment contributing to such deleterious consequences are characterised as a 'malignant social psychology'. They would include treating the person as a child, or as an object, rather than as a person, a human being. Interactions with the person which leave the person outpaced or feeling intimidated or which seek to gain the person's cooperation through deception would similarly be seen as damaging. The overall effect of the malignant social psychology is to devalue, depersonalise and dehumanise the individual with dementia, to diminish and detract from personhood.

Kitwood is careful to emphasise that carers and supporters are not generally malicious in their intent. Rather, dementia seems to attract to itself this type of response. It might be added that these attitudes seem to come to the fore wherever care is provided, whatever the specific condition, and that in the case of dementia or other disorders involving cognitive impairment, the problem arises that the person is particularly unable to resist the impact of the malignant social psychology in ways that are deemed appropriate. The person ultimately has the choice of withdrawing, shutting off from the puzzling, unsupportive environment, or of joining battle using verbal and physical aggression, 'attention-seeking' and other disruptive behaviour, to try to retain a voice in what is happening to them.

The core value that is seen as potentially able to counter the malignant social psychology is to support the personhood of the individual with dementia. Families at times talk of a 'living bereavement', the body remains, but the person has gone. In so doing they are communicating the extent of what has been lost, but while the person will have lost abilities and roles, good dementia care can support the person so that he/she can continue to function as a person. It represents a change of focus, looking not for what was present previously, but for what is present now. All of us change, more or less subtly over the years, and become, in a sense, a different person from that which we were previously. However, we use our memories and our cognitive abilities to maintain a sense of continuity. I cannot become again the person I was ten years ago – that person is effectively 'dead', the clock cannot be turned back. I, together with those who knew me then, can continue to access that time through our collective (not always accurate) memories. I can no longer do some of the things I did then, but there are some new abilities I have acquired over the years. The person with dementia has changed dramatically, but unless we go down the road of only allowing personhood to those with a certain level of cognitive ability, they remain a person. It is not that they are now a part-person; they are indeed a different person from previously (as we all are), needing a lot of support, help and facilitation to maintain the links with their past which their own memory alone may not allow. It is in interaction with the social world that personhood is expressed, and again the help of others is needed to enable its expression to withstand the onslaught of the malignant social psychology, which threatens to overwhelm it. Kitwood has developed a number of indicators of relative well being, ways of identifying the signs of personhood breaking through – social awareness, humour, expressing a wish or desire, for example. Kitwood also suggests that dementia should not simply be seen as an experience of decline, but argues that development may actually be possible. He has collected together reports of people with dementia who have developed new interests, discovered a new creativity, or shown what are perceived to be positive personality changes, despite the presence of a dementia.

For families, and for the person him/herself, there may well be a process of grieving for what is lost; but this is only part of the picture. The current person can be nurtured through good dementia care, and development and growth is by no means impossible. Those around the person can help to maintain links with the past, so that the person does not exist in a vacuum, isolated from what has gone before. A great deal is required of those who provide care to achieve all this, and their support must be a priority also, to ensure that they do have the resources to hold on to the personhood of the individual with dementia, so that he/she is not effectively declared a non-person.

2. EXCESS DISABILITIES

We have already discussed the possibility that certain types of social environment may lead to the person functioning at a lower level than that dictated by the actual damage to brain processes and structures. It is tempting to attribute everything about the person to his/her dementing condition, and to neglect consideration of other factors that may be contributing to the pattern of difficulties observed. This is especially unfortunate, as some of these other factors may be open to amelioration; their recognition and understanding may open the way to improving the situation.

A devaluing, depersonalising social environment is an important, but not the sole, source of excess disability. Others would include:

- *The physical environment*: Most of us have experienced how some buildings are much more confusing and disorientating than others; people with dementia have the same experience – yet more so – and are more disabled in some environments than in others (e.g. Netten 1993). Lack of landmarks and distinctive features, absent or unclear signposting, toilets not clearly marked or easy to access would add to the problems of some people with dementia, for example. Or a busy place, unfamiliar people coming and going, lots of noise, TV and radio blaring out, may stretch the person's ability to process all that is happening to such an extent that an overload panic reaction occurs. A sudden change of environment may be devastating for those whose function has been maintained by familiar cues and automatic patterns of behaviour in a particular place, or by patterns of support and assistance from familiar people. This is why sometimes the first indications of a dementia occur when the person goes away to somewhere unfamiliar on holiday. Admission to a residential or nursing home, or to a respite care unit may similarly lead to a reduction in function, and further excess disability. To assess the person in an unfamiliar environment may give an indication of the potential for dysfunction, but it cannot be the best way of discovering the person's optimal level of function.

- *Physical health*: In the absence of a dementing process, physical health problems can at times lead to delirium or acute confusion, where the person is disorientated with poor concentration and, in many cases, experiences hallucinations. When a dementia is present the person often seems more vulnerable to such reactions, to say a chest or bladder infection. Reactions to drugs – prescribed or non-prescribed – and alcohol may also be important. For instance, in fit healthy young people benzodiazepines (such as diazepam) impair memory – in someone with a significant impairment of memory, the effect could be much greater. Adapting to sensory difficulties – vision and hearing loss – may be more difficult with a coexisting dementia. The person with dementia's physical well being will in any case be more vulnerable, if he/she has difficulty reporting or describing any symptoms experienced, or in complying with necessary, medical treatment or dietary regimes. Thus a person with diabetes may be less able to maintain appropriate blood-sugar levels, and may show additional cognitive impairment from this source.

- *Depression and anxiety*: Relatively large proportions of people with dementia also show features of depression and/or anxiety (Ballard *et al.* 1996; Reifler and Larson 1990). Given the extent of change experienced by the person, and the inherent difficulty in coping with a condition usually involving a progressive reduction in cognitive abilities, this may not be surprising. However, the extent to which the anxiety and depression accompanying dementia reduce function is often not appreciated. As with physical health, it may be less easy for the person with dementia to monitor and report on his/her mood and level of fear, worry and anxiety; often depression and anxiety are not recognised by staff or caregivers. Depression and anxiety may lead to avoidance of activities and interests that might previously have been enjoyed; or to a reluctance to carry out self-care tasks of which he/she was quite capable. As others take over the task in question, the ability is lost, and perhaps never recovered. The person may become restless and nervous, or apparently uncooperative. Some will ask the same question repeatedly, often not waiting for the answer before repeating it again. The desperate search for reassurance takes over, and reduces further the cognitive capacity available for managing daily life.

3. LEARNING IS POSSIBLE

Although it is clear that learning is difficult in dementia, it is important to note that it is not impossible. Whilst many neuropsychological studies in dementia have tended to delineate the areas of deficit, a few have highlighted the conditions under which learning and memory do occur, in younger as well as with older patients (Miller and Morris 1993). One especially interest-ing finding is that once information is learned, rates of forgetting after the first ten minutes or so are relatively normal in dementia. There is also evidence that procedural memory – as seen in the learning of motor skills – is relatively intact. Backman (1992) summarises the research as indicating that the person with dementia needs support at both the time of learning and at the time of retrieval; more learning trials are required, learning fewer items at a time; more assistance is required in encoding the material to be learned, with more cues provided to assist the retrieval process.

4. WORKING WITH SUPPORTERS

Any intervention must consider the needs of those supporting the person with dementia. If they are already experiencing severe strain, expecting them to carry out a demanding programme of activities with the person will be unrealistic. It may be more relevant to consider a stress-management approach aimed directly at their distress, in fact. Family members and friends less immediately involved may be more able to spend time with the person, working on involving the person in purposeful activities. It is also important to select targets for change that will assist the caregivers, as well as improving the quality of life for the person with dementia. Most of the useful work that can be done will need to be long-term, and set in the place where the person spends most time. Engaging in a collaborative relationship with the person and their supporters is essential. Maintaining channels of communication is the key; supporters need assistance to be able to listen, by tuning in as effec- tively as possible to what the person is saying (in words and feelings), as well as learning the most helpful ways of expressing themselves so that the person with dementia is able to understand their meaning as clearly as possible. Good communication is hard work, but it is well worth the effort. Many instances of challenging behaviour, such as aggression, occur because of mis- understood communication. For example, the caregiver is intending to communicate that he/she is going to help the person change out of their soiled clothes, but the message picked up by the person with dementia is one of threat, of someone entering their personal private space without permis- sion; the response is to shout and lash out at the perceived attack. Holden and Woods (1995, Chapter 7) discuss in more detail communication in dementia.

5. AN INDIVIDUALISED APPROACH

Whilst general principles together with a few techniques with a relatively wide applicability can be identified, the reality is that each case is unique, and that only a highly individualised approach has any chance of being useful. The differences come from a variety of sources including:

- the type and subtype of dementia present
- the pattern and trajectory of impairment
- the stage of progression the impairment has reached
- the person's attempts at coping with what is happening (e.g. use of denial, self-blame etc.)
- the person's previous lifestyle, life experiences, abilities and interests
- the support available to the person and his/her relationship with key supporters
- the excess disabilities present.

The information that the person has a diagnosis of dementia is, in itself, remarkably uninformative, and a great deal more information regarding the individual and his/her situation is needed before a care plan can be drawn up. The assessment needs to be thorough and wide ranging and should seek to identify the person's strengths, their areas of retained function and ability, as well as the areas of difficulty where support and help will be needed. Whatever the person's age, the assessment should be placed in the context of their life story to date; what has been important to and valued by the person? What are the key interests, experiences and relationships?

A neuropsychological assessment is essential, covering the range of cognitive abilities at a level appropriate for the person concerned. As well as memory and learning (verbal and non-verbal, immediate and after a delay), this should cover language, perceptual abilities, constructional abilities, speed of processing, reasoning and planning skills (see Davies 1996; Miller and Morris 1993; Morris and McKiernan 1994). Results from such an assessment can be a useful source of feedback for the person and his/her supporters. For instance, understanding that the battles over dressing the person arise not from the person being awkward but from a dressing dyspraxia – a neuropsychological impairment, where the person cannot coordinate their limb and body movements with their intention – can lead to a more constructive approach, and prevent the person being blamed for something outside their own control.

Seeking understanding of behavioural disturbance and difficulty, of 'problem' or 'challenging' behaviour is an essential component of the assessment process. This involves careful detailed description, observation and definition, avoiding generalised terms such as 'attention seeking' or 'wandering' or 'incontinence' which can mean all manner of things (see Stokes 1996). The contribution of the care environment to the problems should be considered particularly carefully, alongside the other causes of excess disability. Many problem behaviours can, without too much of a leap of the imagination, be seen as an understandable attempt by the person to deal with what are for them unprecedentedly difficult circumstances. Frustration and anger at not being able to succeed at tasks previously well within the person's capabilities, or at not being able to understand what is happening, are extreme reactions; the person is in an extreme situation.

In selecting areas to address in a plan of intervention, it is important to select goals that are not only relevant to the person and his/her supporters, but are also attainable. Progress can be made, but the steps will usually be small. All involved need to be able to recognise and value the small changes that are possible – by careful selection of goals, these small changes can be sufficient to make a real difference to the person's quality of life. The process of care planning is ongoing. As the situation changes, new strategies and goals will need to be identified; the future cannot be predicted, but there needs to be sufficient flexibility to allow for the day-to-day changes and fluctuations that are almost inevitable. Maintaining the person's function is a key goal; skills can soon be lost, and supporters need particular help in avoiding 'taking over'. It is tempting when the person is struggling with a task, or taking a long time, to step in and complete it for them. Often there is an assessment of risk to be made; are there other ways of keeping risk to an acceptable level, short of preventing the person engaging in the activity? What level of risk is acceptable? The goal should be to give the person with dementia just enough support and assistance so that they are able to continue to carry out the activities important to them, but in practice this can be a difficult judgement to make. Some guidance for this and other difficult decisions may come from knowledge of the person's previous personality and coping style; if he/she valued independence and control greatly, for example, supporting the person's sense of control and independence should be given priority.

Specific approaches

1. COGNITIVE MANAGEMENT

There is a long-standing literature on the use of 'reality orientation' with people with dementia. In essence, in its purest form, this was a cognitive approach aiming to increase the person's knowledge of and awareness of what was happening around them. The extensive evaluative literature shows clearly that gains in verbal orientation can be achieved through simple repetition and learning techniques (see Holden and Woods 1995; Woods and Roth 1996). More recently, cognitive management techniques have been further refined, and based on more efficient learning methods. For example, there have been several studies demonstrating the potential of spaced-retrieval (Camp *et al.* 1996). Here the person learns one item at a time, with the period between presentation of the item and the request for retrieval being gradually lengthened, as long as the person is able to retrieve the item on each trial. Thus initially it might be one second, then five, then ten, and so on. If the person is unable to recall the item the retrieval period is reduced on the next trial and then built up again when the person is able to retrieve it at the shorter period again. It has been suggested that errorless learning may be especially useful in dementia, where incorrect answers have the potential to interfere with what is being learned. Thus, if we make a mistake over someone's name, the next time we meet we may have difficulty disentangling which was the correct name and which was the incorrect name we mistakenly used last time. All we can remember is that it was a problem! By discouraging the person from guessing, building up slowly the retrieval time and providing ample retrieval cues, errorless learning can be attempted with people with dementia.

Such methods may be used, for example, to teach the person to use a memory aid, such as a calendar, diary or notebook, which can then help to relieve the load on memory. They might also be used to help the person remember a particularly important piece of information. Thus, if a person asks a question repeatedly due to a memory problem, it may be worth using this strategy to help them recall the answer for themselves (see Camp *et al.* 1996 for an example of this).

2. BEHAVIOURAL MANAGEMENT

Examples of behavioural approaches in dementia are relatively rare in practice. As well as its cognitive component, reality orientation included components of behavioural training. Thus there are a number of reports of people with dementia learning their way around an environment, using signposts provided, with simple, repetitive training (see Holden and Woods 1995). Other examples are in relation to self-care (e.g. Josephsson *et al.* 1993; Pinkston and Linsk 1984), mobility (Burgio *et al.* 1986), social interaction (Bourgeois 1990; Green, Linsk and Pinkston 1986), and continence (Burgio *et al.* 1988; Schnelle *et al.* 1993). Most commonly, it is the prompting element of the intervention that seems particularly useful. Indeed in some of the studies (specifically those on mobility and continence) gains have been so rapid that no learning mechanism can have been operating. The environment had previously simply not provided prompting of appropriate behaviour, resulting in excess disability.

The most promising work to date on behaviour problems comes from Australia, where Bird, Alexopoulos and Adamowicz (1995) report a number of individual case studies illustrating an individualised approach to their management, making extensive use of retrieval cues. The association between the cue and the desired response is taught intensively using the cognitive methods described above. Thus a person who repeatedly went, mistakenly, into other people's rooms learned that a sign outside these rooms meant she was not to enter. Another person who repeatedly asked to go to the toilet for fear of an accident, learnt to go when a buzzer sounded, set at intervals appropriate to her need for urination. Woods and Bird (1998) report further examples, including interventions for inappropriate sexual behaviour.

3. EMOTIONAL MANAGEMENT

One of the developments in dementia care over the last few years has been the rediscovery of the emotional life of the person with dementia. From the moment of diagnosis (indeed, from the beginning of the diagnostic assessment process) the person's emotional response to what is happening is a vital element, influencing quality of life, coping attempts, behavioural disturbance and the whole caregiving process.

The first intervention in this sphere will be *de facto* the manner in which the diagnosis is (or, more usually, is not) shared with the patient (Rice and Warner 1994). Relatives may prefer the patient not to be told, but in so doing they operate a double standard, as they state clearly they would want to be told if they were the patient (Maguire *et al.* 1996). Good practice should be to engage in prediagnostic counselling, to explore and clarify what should be told to whom. It is not simply the name of the condition that might be shared, of course. It is the implications – for work, for relationships, for children, for driving, for the future – that really matter. The implications need to be separated out clearly from any preconceived ideas the person may have regarding the condition from the media, from other experiences and so on. Some patients will cope with the situation by denial, and will need time and space to absorb their experience, as they seek to protect the integrity of their current self-concept. Others will minimise the problems; others will see a conspiracy, blaming others for making up stories about them; others still will feel devastation and despair. The scope for psychological therapy has been recognised, with several accounts of psychodynamic therapy (e.g. Hausman 1992; Sinason 1992) and of cognitive behaviour therapy in relation to depression (Teri and Gallagher-Thompson 1991; Thompson *et al.* 1990).

Validation therapy (Feil 1993) has emphasised the emotional world of the person with dementia, and offers some useful techniques for communication at the emotional level, tuning in to the feelings and meanings behind the words which are spoken. Resolution therapy (Stokes and Goudie 1990) proposes an empathic listening approach, with similar intent. Validation has tended to be associated with an unnecessarily complex theoretical background, with more emphasis on unresolved memories from the person's life than on current difficulties. The common ground appears to be in the importance of listening to the person's emotional expression, without getting enmeshed in facts, dates and current reality; entering into the person's world, seeking to understand from his/her perspective, rather than imposing our own reality. The value of engaging in this work early so that the therapist is able to make sense of later, less clearly articulated communication, is demonstrated by Mills' (1997) account of the change in the person's self-narrative as the disorder progresses.

Reminiscence and life-review work has often been used with older patients as a way of maintaining self-narrative, the person's story of their life (Gibson 1994). Younger people similarly reminisce, particularly at times of change, and so this may prove a useful technique in this context also, as part of the therapeutic work. Life-story books have been used with people of all ages, to assist in maintaining a sense of self in rapidly changing circumstances. Outside the therapeutic context, it can also prove an enjoyable social activity; maintaining social contact will for many be an important part of preserving self-esteem. Small groups, purposeful and interesting activities and building on the familiar assist in enabling the person to continue social roles. The person does not have to enter a different world, but adaptations may be needed to allow him/her to function in previous roles. Thus the person might still visit the same pub, but now with one or two friends only, instead of a large group, and at a quieter time. Alcohol intake might also need to be reduced!

A number of 'therapies' are attracting interest at present, for example aromatherapy, therapeutic massage, and Snoezelen (Baker *et al.* 1997;

Brooker *et al.* 1997; Spaull, Leach and Frampton 1998). The latter involves gentle music, interesting visual effects, and tactile stimulation. Generally the aim seems to be to encourage relaxation and reduce tension, which is a worthwhile aim for many people with dementia. There is some evidence that relaxation therapy is itself helpful (Welden and Yesavage 1982). Such approaches are unlikely to be universally useful, but are worth considering as

---

Case study: John

John G, 56 years, was on referral to the memory clinic living with his wife and two teenage children. Two years previously he and his wife had been referred elsewhere for family therapy, as he had been accusing his wife of having an affair with a good-looking young man living nearby. They had separated for a time, but the delusional jealousy receded when the young man moved away. For his wife, the diagnosis of dementia was almost a relief after the hurt and distress of the previous few years, where she had borne the brunt of her husband's morbid jealousy, which had made her question the many years of happy marriage they had enjoyed previously. Now she could attribute the problems to the developing dementia, and at last felt that she knew what she was coping with. The teenage children spent a lot of time away from home, but wanted to support their mother as much as possible. John admitted that his memory was not as good as it was, but generally made light of the difficulties. However, he could no longer carry on with his work, and this added a financial pressure to the family's situation.

John was involved in family meetings about the future and the family's needs as far as he was able. Finding activities for John to occupy his time was seen as a priority by his wife, and she was able to involve him in an adaptation of his previous interest in art – colouring in ready-drawn pictures, as he was no longer able to create a picture himself. Aggressive outbursts became a problem; these were tackled by Mrs G learning to identify particular precipitants and developing strategies for avoiding these. Mrs G attends a carers' support group, where she has helped other carers to develop coping strategies as well as receiving support herself. Respite care has been considered, but, like many of the services offered, would have involved John in a setting with much older people. The alternative, of having someone come to spend time with John at home, encouraging his art and other hobbies, has proved more acceptable to John and his family.

a relatively safe alternative to the use of tranquillisers to assist the person to be less tense and anxious.

Conclusion

The potential for psychosocial interventions with younger people with dementia is clear, but there is an urgent need for work specifically addressing the needs of such individuals. The growing awareness of the issues around sharing the diagnosis and of the significance of the emotional response of the person with dementia to their condition could lead to valuable developments. Professionals must listen, carefully, sensitively, respectfully, empathically to the person with dementia as well as to their supporters. They will then be in a better position to negotiate with the person and their care givers appropriate strategies of intervention and support. There is a growing range of options available from work with older adults; with creativity and empathy the possibility exists with younger people also of reducing excess disability and of supporting the person with dementia through whatever their condition may bring.

CHAPTER 15

Support Groups for People with Early Stage Alzheimer's Disease

Robyn Yale

Introduction

> It helps to know you aren't alone – listening to how others deal with similar problems… it makes me feel much better to know that there are people like me…

This statement speaks to the power support groups have to assist people in coping with specific difficulties. It could be describing a group focused on, for example, surviving cancer, abstaining from alcohol, or caring for a relative with a chronic illness. This was said, however, by someone in a group for individuals with early stage Alzheimer's disease (AD). These were patients *of all ages* who were seeking information and support while only mildly impaired by the illness.

The mental health needs of this unique and newly recognised subpopulation have been seriously overlooked and underserved. As early detection methods improve, and as concerns mount about incidence, costs and consequences of the disease, this gap in the continuum of dementia care has become glaringly apparent. The intervention described herein targets the lack of attention to those who have AD, and to the issues which make the beginning stages of the illness unique for these patients and their families.

This chapter describes a research study which documents themes and interactions in a support group for individuals with early stage AD. The voices of the participants convey a compelling message. Early dementia is characterised not only by impairments which have become perceptible, but by abilities remaining intact as well. Each person responds differently to the dawning awareness of difficulties and newly required adjustments. While some cope by denying their condition, others are willing and able to talk about the disease, and display an amazing resilience and determination in the face of it.

This research study was intended as a stepping stone to making support services for early AD patients much more widely available. Hopefully, the results will help to demystify discussion of the AD diagnosis, and desensitise those who may be interested in but fearful of talking with patients about the illness. The intervention has since been refined and systematised, and step-by-step guidelines for developing this type of support group are available (Yale 1995).

Clarifying the terms 'Early Stage' and 'Early Onset' AD

Clarification of the difference between 'early stage' and 'early onset' AD is useful here. Early stage refers to a person with dementia who is only mildly impaired, regardless of their current age. Early onset refers to a person with dementia who is under 65 years of age, regardless of their current level of impairment.

For example, early stage AD individuals of any age (who are within the beginning range of disease progression) are likely to experience significant disruptions and challenges in such areas as work, activities, and family relationships. However, they are typically self-aware, able to live and manage personal care independently, and have relatively good communication skills. For those with early dementia who plateau or progress slowly, there may be many years ahead of good health and high functioning before there is further decline.

On the other hand, early onset AD individuals (younger than age 65) may have mild, moderate or severe cognitive and functional impairment – as may people over age 65. Only those in the early stages would be appropriate for the type of support group discussed here. Since AD affects each individual differently, neither age nor time since onset/diagnosis alone can predict the ability to effectively participate in this intervention. The most important criteria for group selection, then, are level of impairment along with the degree of openness and acceptance of the disease.

Commonalities between younger and older individuals with early stage AD

The participants in this particular early stage support group spanned a range of ages. The average age was 68 (three participants were between 56 and 60 years of age; and four were between 71 and 79 years old). The author's experience with this and subsequent groups has been that age has never presented a barrier in terms of either relevant topics or the quality of relationships between group members. Generally, older and younger people with mild dementia do well together in groups. They are primarily relieved to meet one another and have the group setting, as they forge a common bond in facing and coping with AD.

You will see from the themes and interactions detailed on pages 276–279, for example, that individuals of mixed ages with early dementia were dealing with the trauma of emotional adjustments and disruptions in identity, abilities, lifestyle and relationships. People often have similar feelings, concerns, and experiences to share regardless of how old they are when they develop dementia.

Issues unique to younger individuals with early stage AD

As the larger context of this book focuses on the younger person with dementia, it is important to identify any issues that are unique to individuals with early AD who are below age 65. Having discussed above the themes common between younger and older patients, the major distinction to make regards the younger person's earlier point in the life span, and the resulting implications.

Younger people are often in the midst of careers and raising their own families when symptoms of AD begin. While older people with early dementia can also be living full and active lives, the developmental tasks and expectations are different in mid-life. (This is more applicable, though, between two people who are 54 and 84 years old, for example, than between two who are 62 and 66 years old.)

Anecdotal generalisations from younger AD patients in support groups relay the shock of becoming cognitively impaired at the workplace. Eventual diagnosis of AD often leads to retirement many years before one would expect this to happen – dramatically affecting self-esteem, lifestyle and the whole area of finances. Previous plans for the years after retirement may become a fading dream, given the probability of future decline by the time of older age. The spouse of a younger individual with AD is suddenly the sole breadwinner and gradually the manager of all household responsibilities. The AD patient, meanwhile, is experiencing losses uncharacteristic of this age range, including changes in family roles, identity and driving privileges.

New ways to spend time and feel productive are necessary, typically without friends who are in the same situation. Unexpected dependency on spouses and children due to AD is a struggle, and affects the capacity to be a partner or parent in all the ways that were established and anticipated for years to come. Furthermore, younger people with AD often have young or young adult children who must cope emotionally and/or as caregivers very early in their own lives. (Thus, services for children of people with AD are also needed.)

Over time, the patient may 'miss' important life events such as becoming a grandparent or witnessing the success of a child's endeavours. Also, younger people with AD may have their own ageing parents alive; another way in which AD is 'out of sync' at this stage of life. While the challenge of anyone with early stage AD is to accept and adjust to the disease, the younger patient must do so when many years of life are potentially ahead.

Services for family members of people with early stage AD

Family members of all individuals with early stage AD have issues that are unique from those caring for more impaired people. Early on, families are newly learning about the disease, making adjustments, and sorting out the patients' impairments and abilities. It is often difficult to know how much autonomy the patient is capable of vs. how much supervision is needed, and to take on this unfamiliar caregiving role. Page 273 relays some concerns of early stage caregivers in the study, and younger spouses and children additionally deal with the issues described above.

Since the time of this research, a concurrent, separate group for family members of the early stage AD support group participants has been added as a beneficial programme component. The joint experience of going to separate groups allows both patients and families to each talk with others in similar situations. It is hoped that this also facilitates communication between them at home about important emotional and planning matters.

An adaptable, replicable model

The early stage AD support group model described is replicable and adaptable to people younger than 65, older than 65, and a mixed range of ages. The opportunity to talk about and learn to cope with AD provides the same potential benefits to group members of all ages. The major criteria for group participation have to do with ability and willingness, regardless of age. Both common and unique themes between age groups have been addressed, but one must not overgeneralise. Each patient is an individual, and deserves assessment of the impact of AD on their own life circumstances.

Many agencies just beginning to develop early stage services initially make them available to everyone. Deciding upon a target population within a region ultimately depends on the community need that emerges as well as the goals and resources of the service provider. Ideally, support groups offer a therapeutic environment for early stage AD patients in which they can receive: (a) information about the disease after diagnosis; (b) emotional support; (c) help with problem-solving; (d) ideas about needs in the future; and (e) encouragement to continue living well and fully in the present.

Research summary: Support groups for newly diagnosed, early stage Alzheimer's patients – how patients manage their concerns

This study was funded by a Pilot Research Grant from the National Alzheimer's Association and conducted (1992) at University of California, San Francisco by: Joseph Barbaccia, MD, Principal Investigator; Linda Mitteness, PhD, Co-Principal Investigator; Robyn Yale, LCSW, Project Director; and Catherine Lee, MA, Research Assistant.

Research questions

> I felt really good doing something for myself – I've gotten so much out of it. It may be helpful for my wife too – she knows I'm trying... I'm not a quitter!

This study explored how patients with early dementia respond to a professionally led peer support group focused on understanding and coping with AD. Research questions included:

1. Can early dementia patients express their concerns about AD in a support group?

2. Will these concerns change after the intervention and several months later?

3. Will the support group affect the emotional health and social functioning of these patients?

4. Will patients' participation in a support group affect the level of burden in their caregivers?

Procedures

Fifteen early AD patients and their caregivers were assigned to either treatment or control conditions. The treatment consisted of eight weekly group meetings for the patients only, focused on education and support around the illness. Group sessions were observed, documented and analysed. The 'controls' received only usual care (in the settings from which they were referred) during this period, and were offered a patient support group when data collection was completed. All patients and their caregivers were interviewed at three points in time: before and after the intervention, and an average of two months later. The third interview with all study participants concluded with an offer of general consultation and referral to appropriate community resources.

The sample

Since the manifestation and course of AD differs for each patient, the distinction of 'newly diagnosed' did not turn out to be a useful one. The target population was redefined as 'early stage', as determined by mild impairment on cognitive testing and interview responses. A score of 18-24 on the Mini-Mental Status Exam (Folstein, Folstein and McHugh 1975) was used as one selection criterion.

Only patients who had been told that they probably had Alzheimer's disease (by a physician and/or family member), at least occasionally acknowledged their memory loss, could potentially communicate their feelings and experiences about the illness, and were willing and able to give informed consent could participate in the study. All patients had a documented diagnosis of probable or possible AD most recently evaluated within the previous approximate two years, and three had additional dementia-related diagnoses. None had other significant medical or psychiatric conditions. Each patient had a family caregiver who was willing to be interviewed and with whom contact occurred at least several times weekly.

Participants were recruited through media coverage as well as referrals from the many Alzheimer's service providers in the San Francisco Bay Area. While 76 inquiries were received initially, only 15 patients were subsequently enrolled. Study inclusion criteria were not met in most instances. For example, approximately 1/3 of those who were interested in the support group were inquiring on behalf of a patient who was either too cognitively impaired to participate and/or was likely to have behavioral or social difficulties in the group. Over 1/5 of the calls concerned patients who had either not been told – or were told but denied – their diagnosis. In these instances, where caregivers wanted patients to participate so they would 'face and accept' their condition, it was explained that this was not the project's intent.

Contact with the project was initiated in some cases by patients themselves who had learned of the study through newspaper articles. In all cases, caregivers provided historical information during a telephone screening and intake process. Staff then spoke briefly to the patient on the phone to explain the study, assess initial comprehension and interest, and seek permission to set up an enrollment interview. Consent was secured for the patients' medical records to be reviewed by the principal investigator. Interviews with those eligible were held by two staff who met with each patient and caregiver jointly and then separately in the home or research office.

Patients were assigned to either a treatment or control group based on such factors as transportation and scheduling constraints, rather than by their characteristics or abilities. Study participants were diverse in age, gender, ethnicity, and family constellation. A final sample of thirteen completed the project: seven in the support and six in the control group.

The intervention

The intervention consisted of eight weekly support group sessions of 1.5 hours' duration. The group was facilitated by the project director (a licensed clinical social worker), who had previously developed a training manual for leaders of patient support groups.

A circle of chairs 'set the stage' for the meetings. The facilitator reviewed the purpose and ground rules at the start of each session, providing structure and direction while encouraging group decision-making and monitoring participation. Discussion was kept as focused and uncomplicated as possible by raising one issue at a time and continually clarifying and reframing main points. Topics were suggested by the facilitator but increasingly initiated by patients over time. Examples of themes, such as adapting to cognitive loss and changes in family relationships, will be elaborated in the 'Results' section.

Patients were amazingly able to raise difficult issues, share their feelings, 'educate' one another, and commit themselves to the project goals. While interaction between members was fostered, each patient's style and boundaries were also respected. For example, patients in periodic denial were not forcefully confronted. Overall, because participants were carefully screened before enrollment and welcomed the opportunity to discuss the illness, the need for the facilitator to intervene was less than had been anticipated.

Techniques used by the facilitator accommodated patients' cognitive impairments. For example, forgetfulness which occurred within the group was attributed to the disease process, identified as common amongst group members, and compared to problems occurring outside of the group as well (e.g., 'What do you do in other situations when you have trouble finding a word?'). Patients having difficulty expressing themselves were asked whether they wanted assistance and if so, the facilitator restated, interpreted, and checked the accuracy of what was intuited. Patients' abilities as well as their limitations were acknowledged (e.g., 'You seem able to communicate well in the group – what can help you do that when stressful situations come up elsewhere?').

Patients were brought to the meetings and picked up by their caregivers, who often congregated and chatted informally while waiting. The caregivers attended the last session to discuss the group with patients and staff, exchange names and phone numbers, and say good-bye to one another.

Data collection and analysis

Study data consisted of interviews, documentation of support group sessions, and evaluation of the group experience:

1. Three interviews were conducted separately with all patients and care-givers: at enrollment (T1), after the eight-week support group period (T2), and an average of two months later (T3). It was not possible to un-earth any existing measurement tools which assessed status or pin-pointed concerns specific to early stage AD. Therefore, validated instruments were supplemented by clinical interviews constructed by the research team.

    Patients were assessed at all three points in time on the Mini-Mental Status Exam (Folstein, Folstein and McHugh 1975) and the Global Deterioration Scale (Reisberg *et al.* 1982) to determine the level of cognitive impairment; and on the Hamilton Rating Scale for Depression (Hamilton 1960). A semi-structured questionnaire based on the domains of the Linn Social Dysfunctioning Rating Scale (Linn *et al.* 1969) was administered, which covered mood, changes in social relationships and activity level, and patients' perceptions of, adjustments to and concerns about their condition.

Caregivers were administered scales of depression and burden using a subset of the Stress and Coping Interview (Pearlin *et al.* 1990). Other interview questions developed by the research team covered caregivers' perceptions of patients' reactions to the illness; and the impact of the illness on the patients' and families' lives.

2. Support group sessions were observed by a trained research assistant and audiotaped to capture themes and interactions. A specific format was developed to document the process of the group as a whole and record each participant's affect, behaviour and nonverbal communication at every meeting. Areas covered included topics initiated by patients, emotions expressed, levels of participation, and interpersonal styles.

3. Patients who were in the support group were asked to evaluate the group at T2. Caregivers of these participants were asked for their impressions of patients' responses to the group experience at T2 and T3.

Study data were by the co-principal investigator using both quantitative and qualitative techniques. Examination of the established assessment scales followed the model of a repeated measures analysis of variance. Due to the small sample size, only large differences between treatment and control groups were found to be significant. Results of these statistical analyses need to be interpreted with caution in light of the small sample size, and are, therefore, supplemented with a focus on the specific responses of patients and caregivers.

Interviews and support group observations were subjected to limited (primarily nonparametric) statistical analyses, and were categorized using standard qualitative methods. Coding strategies were first developed by the whole research team and thus interobserver reliability was established before any responses were coded. A sequential data analysis model was then used looking first for similarities and patterns within groups, then for changes over time and finally, for differences between groups.

Results

1. INTERVIEWS WITH EARLY STAGE PATIENTS AND CAREGIVERS

(i) Patients' concerns: Patients were willing and able to discuss the impact of memory loss and their feelings about it in interviews. Patients described an awareness of inabilities to do things they had always done, and concerns about problems they might eventually develop. Most were able to identify

specific areas of difficulty. For example, one knew that: 'Remembering words is the problem… If I try to give an answer immediately I can't do it – I need time.' Another remarked, 'I get frustrated when I'm with too many people at once – I can't get the fun they are having and feel very bad about that.'

Patients had varying degrees of acceptance of the changes in their lives. At one end of the spectrum was the person who explained, 'I look at it philosophically – everyone's going to die and doesn't know how it will happen… if I didn't have AD it might be something else'. Another expressed a different viewpoint: 'I feel angry – why me??! I can't do the things I used to do.' When asked whether they worry about anything in particular, one patient admitted, 'I don't think I'll ever go back to how I was and it scares me. I wish I could do something about it.'

The experiences of being interviewed and attending a support group seemed to make patients feel understood and therefore able to 'do something about it.' For example, one concluded the first interview on a note of hope and determination, exclaiming, 'I feel better already – I feel I can do this!'

Patients in the support group were found to be more likely than controls to discuss problems related to their illness. Support group patients were also more likely than controls to acknowledge that their diagnosis was AD when asked at the second interview, and were significantly more open about AD with their caregivers at this point in time than they had been initially. In contrast, only one control patient had discussed and made plans around AD at the time of second interview. By the third interview, several patients who had been in the support group were seeking information about other dementia-related services, such as day programmes and individual therapy specific to AD.

(ii) Caregivers' perceptions of patients' concerns: Caregivers described major changes in patients' social lives, work lives, relationships, and identities: 'He was always an active scientist and intellectual, and is no longer capable of that. An entire reassessment of himself and his future was necessary.' Many previous activities had been effected by the illness: 'Socializing has decreased …he never wants to go out. He feels self-conscious, that he won't know how to interact with friends anymore.'

Caregivers sensed that patients had mixed feelings about the explanation for their symptoms. One noted some positive aspects: 'Sometimes he feels the loss; yet, there's also relief [about the diagnosis] because things have been effortful for years without knowing why. He's now happier, more relaxed, and more emotionally available.' Another commented on her relative's lone-liness: 'She'd like to do more [socially] but she's unsure of herself – she's scared that she won't be able to make herself understood.'

Several caregivers mentioned that they had discussed worries about the future with patients, as increasing cognitive and functional impairment became more apparent: 'He's appropriately concerned – he worries what will happen if he becomes unable to talk.' Some had agreed together on prefer-ences for long-term care arrangements: 'He's concerned about me [wife] – working too hard... He asked me to promise that I would place him in a nurs-ing home if he later becomes a burden for me.'

(iii) Caregivers' concerns: When asked about changes which were newly trou-blesome for themselves, caregivers identified shifting roles and relationships with patients: 'I'm now the only breadwinner and caretaker... ours was a very equitable relationship, we always made joint decisions after lengthy dis-cussion – I miss this interaction.' Loss of intimacy was mentioned by some of the caregivers as well: 'There have been sexual changes. Sex is less frequent and she is fearful of it.'

Caregivers related other stresses such as isolation, the need for respite, and lack of family consensus around care needs. The patients' dependency and resistance were also reported as difficult at times. One example was hav-ing to talk to the person differently: 'I have lots of frustration around the constant need for clarification and repetition – I feel angry and then feel bad about that.' Another illustrated with, 'She is more oppositional when you try to help her with things, which exasperates me.'

A few of the caregivers who had themselves attended community support groups felt that their needs were different than those of individuals caring for later stage patients. One caregiver stated strongly that none of the existing lit-erature or services she'd encountered addressed early AD in terms of 'constructing a life, grieving and going on – rather than just dealing with the long-term picture.'

2. ASSESSMENT OF PATIENTS AND CAREGIVERS

(i) Patient status: Generally speaking, assessment data did not indicate statisti-cally significant differences between those patients who were in a support group and those who were not. However, it is difficult to know whether this speaks to the effect of the intervention, the imprecision of existing measure-ment tools, the impact of small sample size on statistical analyses, or a

combination of these and other factors. This is one reason that the study was set up with a process-oriented emphasis, focusing less on outcomes and more on the patients' abilities and responses in the support group. For the sake of completion, data on the cognitive, emotional and social functioning of patients are, however, reported here and should be interpreted with caution as previously stated.

Patients in both treatment and control groups had mean scores representing mild cognitive impairment on the Mini-Mental State Exam and Global Deterioration Scale. All remained within this range over time, although there was some individual decline within each group. Improvement had not been expected amongst support group participants, given that all AD patients decline cognitively at an unpredictable but continuous rate.

None of the individual or mean scores for either group, at any of the measurement times, reached significance for clinical depression as measured by the Hamilton Rating Scale. The impact of group participation on patients' emotional health was difficult to evaluate, however, particularly since several were reacting to other crises (e.g. death of friends/relatives) at T2. Overall, the patients in the support group were neither significantly more distressed, worried or sad (after learning more about the effects of AD, after the end of their group experience); nor were they significantly more cheerful, happy or calm (after sharing experiences with others, knowing they weren't alone). Patients stated that their self-esteem was higher as a result of support group participation, and reported such mood-related benefits as, 'It took away the embarrassment. It made me feel more hopeful, hearing how people cope; knowing you have plenty of options.'

There were no significant changes over time in either group's social functioning in terms of leisure activity level, paid or volunteer work, or relationships. Friends and family were among the topics discussed within support group sessions, though. For example, one patient who was sad that he rarely saw his friends since the onset of AD decided to set up special one-to-one visits with them, after coming to understand that socializing with several people at once increased his confusion.

Patients in the support group reported enjoying each other and described a sense of belonging, but did not consider the group to be a social activity. At the time of third interview, most of these patients recalled and wanted to continue the group experience, while most of the controls were still feeling isolated and had not done much to address the illness.

(ii) Caregiver status: Caregivers in treatment and control groups were assessed as relatively equal in terms of their own emotional status, reporting moderate levels of anger expressed, anxiety, depression, and general overload. Scores on these scales were not significantly different between groups nor did they change significantly over time. However, it was difficult to determine the effect of patient support group participation on caregiver burden, particularly since several caregivers reported dealing with other crises (e.g., moving) at T2. While one could speculate that caregiver stress might be reduced by improvement in patient wellbeing, this is quite difficult to quantify and measure.

Caregivers did describe the patients' support group experience as helpful to their relatives as well as to themselves. When asked at T2 whether there had been any effect on how they felt or the way they did things, one caregiver stated, 'I used to feel guilty [because I had my own activities] ... I felt good that my husband was participating in something that he saw as his. It helped me to know that he was trying to deal with the illness; he had a place he could talk to others.' Several caregivers mentioned having learned about other available services: 'My husband said one group member did volunteer work in an Alzheimer day programme – he was interested in that kind of [social/recreational] opportunity – do you have information on this?' For the daughter of one participant, the group provided a break from caregiving responsibilities. And another caregiver explained the benefit of the group for the whole family: 'My mother is more confident and less anxious about her condition. The group brought things into the open, which was a great relief – now there's less mystery around discussing the disease at home.' Finally, one caregiver felt less isolated after her relative's experience: 'Even though the group wasn't for me it helped to meet other patients and caregivers – most people don't know what we're going through; any connections or understanding I get helps.'

3. SUPPORT GROUP – CONTENT AND PROCESS

(i) Content of patients' concerns in group: Patients in the support group had the motivation and capacity to articulate their questions, experiences, emotions and coping strategies. Topics ranged widely and commonalities among group members emerged immediately. For example, one person discovered in the first meeting that he was not the only one who had had his driving privileges revoked. All of the others had also dealt with this. While some had resigned to accept it, a few had attempted to appeal the action. Several knew

the state law around dementia and driving and were able to explain it to those less familiar with it. Patients also raised early on their awareness of the stereotyped image of a person with AD, and expressed hope that they could challenge the stigma of 'becoming an imbecile' by participating in this research project. Patients balanced humour and optimism about their current wellness with acknowledging everyday frustrations and the uncertainty of the future. Major themes are summarized below to illustrate the nature and depth of discussion.

(a) Diagnosis of AD: How AD is diagnosed and distinguished from normal memory loss; what it was like to experience diagnostic testing (e.g., felt like a child, felt 'dumb' going through it) and to realize the extent of one's impairments in this setting; general questions about the cause and course of the disease.

(b) Stigma: Awareness that AD patients are often perceived as 'six feet under already'; erroneous assumptions that patients will be more physically and mentally incapacitated than they are; others often do things for patients that they can do themselves.

(c) Changes in lifestyle/abilities: Adjusting to having one's career end prematurely; difficulty with speaking, writing, adding numbers, getting lost; using coping strategies (e.g., 'word substitution').

(d) Driving: Reasons for and reactions to having driving privileges revoked; legal and safety concerns around dementia and driving; loss of independence that results from giving up licence.

(e) Dependency: Getting used to needing assistance from others (e.g. with transportation); the struggle to accept help but function as independently as possible; changes in established marital roles (e.g. wife newly managing all finances).

(f) Family: Concern that family members don't understand certain behaviours are due to the illness (e.g. 'I wish my wife would see that I don't do these things on purpose – I'm doing my best – sometimes, she yells at me'); patients are cognizant of the strain on family members who must repeat themselves and try various ways to communicate ('it's not that I'm ignoring her'); patients' love for their family members and deep appreciation for the care provided to them.

(g) Friends: The loss that is felt when friends 'disappear' because they can no longer relate to patients; the need to educate friends who are fearful or misinformed about AD, and to structure comfortable visits; the difficulty when friends expect patients to be worse than they are, or conversely, when friends minimize what patients are going through (in an effort to be supportive).

(h) Communication: Becomes easier when things are slowed down and simplified, and conversely is more difficult with more people and stimuli; patients can let others know what works and what doesn't in this regard; the need for patients to expect less from themselves in this area.

(i) AD research: Interest in current research being done (e.g. medications); great frustration that research has not yet produced a cure for AD; satisfaction that they were offering new information and potentially helping others through participation in this study.

(j) Wellness and optimism: Patients' realization that they may live for many years, with an unpredictable rate of disease progression; the idea of not dwelling on the future, but rather taking it 'a day at a time'; the importance of pleasurable activities and support systems.

(k) Preparing for the future: The necessity of advance legal planning; local AD resources available and services patients (and their families) have utilized; the importance of discussing the illness with family and friends.

(l) The group: The benefit of having the group as a place to learn and talk about AD; the hope that other groups will be developed for other AD patients; reviewing and ending this group experience.

(ii) Observations of patients' interactions in group: Patients became cohesive from the start of meetings and were very engaging, open and supportive with one another. They assisted each other in specific subject areas as well as with such incidents as helping a frailer member into her seat, or suggesting that an individual with hearing loss use a sign saying 'LOUDER, PLEASE' as needed.

Group members treated each other with tolerance and kindness, particularly in regards to difficulty with either cognitive or emotional expression. They became increasingly relaxed and self-disclosing over time. Conversation was sustained, and all of the patients participated although, as might be expected, some were more verbal than others. Patients were cooperative with the facilitator and needed less direction after the first few sessions. While they were willing to discuss difficult issues and feelings, they also respected one anothers' limits. For instance, one patient's initial denial around her deficits eventually subsided after being gently approached by others but left intact (e.g., 'I see, maybe you don't have the same problems as us…but why are you coming here, then?').

Affect was appropriately responsive and varied – at some times serious, pensive and realistic; at other times hopeful and upbeat. Nonverbal behavior usually reflected interest, as in leaning forward or looking at each other when speaking. Humour and good-natured banter occurred often, as illustrated by comments like 'We're getting so comfortable here, soon we'll be borrowing money from each other!' and 'Oh sure you'll remember what you were about to say – I've heard that one before!'

Although the ability of AD patients to retain group support has been questioned, there were obvious indications that participants recalled and valued the experience. For example, they appeared glad to see each other and many greeted one another by name each week. Interestingly, most patients also chose to sit in the same seat for every meeting, and absences of members were always noticed. Finally, anecdotes relevant to previous sessions were often shared (e.g., 'I felt better after we talked about driving and I held on to this all week to tell you: my wife had trouble parking the car one day – I had to do it for her!').

Overall, group members helped each other explore and come to terms with what they were facing, as illustrated by the following:

(a) Examples of patients sharing understanding/knowledge about AD:

> It's important that we all stay healthy – many AD patients die of other illnesses, like pneumonia.

> The reason you have trouble writing [like I do] is because the brain cells aren't connecting to your hand when you need them to.

> I'm like you – when I'm pressured, electric currents go every which way and I lose it completely. In fact, that's what happened in the [diagnostic testing], and they concluded I had AD.

> What is this experimental medication you're on – can I get in on that research too?

> I volunteer at a day center for AD patients – I enjoy helping with the meals and activities they have…

> If your sister doesn't understand you, she could go to a support group – they have them for what they now call 'caregivers'.

(b) Examples of sharing feelings/experiences with one another:

> Am I the only one who hates the word Alzheimer's?

> Do you have this problem too [reading, speaking, etc.]?

> I'm getting used to the idea that I might get worse – I didn't accept it before, but I'm starting to see some changes. Psychologically it seems useful to come to terms with this – what do others of you think?

> I'm not sure what to say – I've lost the thought...[another patient] that's okay – that happens to me a lot!

(c) Examples of sharing perspectives on the illness:

> When you think about the people who were in the Oakland hills fire or the LA riots, you have to admit that we're better off than they are – things could be worse.

> It's been a big adjustment and loss not being able to work anymore. But it's important to find new things to do and enjoy – if you just give up, it's like wanting to die. Your mood can help you get used to the changes.

> Now I realize I do have a problem, but I'm not alone. It's not the end of the world – you've found a way to go on with your lives.

4. PATIENTS' AND CAREGIVERS' RESPONSES TO PATIENTS' GROUP EXPERIENCE

(i) Patients' evaluation of group; Patients generally had positive responses to the group experience and most could identify specific topics which they found helpful to discuss. Only one member, who was in a convalescent facility after knee surgery and was more confused than other patients at T2, had difficulty remembering her group experience. Patients described what they enjoyed about the group at the second interview:

> It's okay to share feelings – I don't talk much usually, I hold inside too much. This helped me try to make my wife understand me.

> I liked not being embarrassed to speak up about things I couldn't [describe] before. And everybody understood, had the same ideas and feelings.

> It helped me a lot to organize my thoughts. The feeling of the group was very positive.

Patients had a sense of altruism and accomplishment about attending the group:

> I felt good about myself for talking, making new friends.

> I felt good that maybe I was able to help others too… I pushed the fact that everyone should go to an attorney for advice.

Patients stated that they felt comfortable with and close to the other group members:

> I felt decent and supported. I won't be going to movies with them, but it was important to do what we did: come in, speak with people and go out. It never occurred to me to do something with them [other than be in group], yet there was not one negative idea.

> My wife and I developed a relationship with Mr H and his wife – they are very fine people. His diagnosis was just this past January, while mine was several years ago!

None of the patients mentioned anything that made them uncomfortable, and all expressed a desire to continue in a group. They were surprised and frustrated at the lack of similar services available in the region. One put it this way: 'My wife is always going to caregiver groups – this one was needed for us!'

(ii) Caregivers' perceptions of patients' group experience. Caregivers reported that patients generally seemed excited each week about the upcoming meeting, and made positive comments about the group. One caregiver said that her husband would not discuss the content of the meetings with her because, he explained, what went on in them was confidential. Most caregivers, however, stated that patients talked about specific topics discussed, liked other group members, and had feelings of relief and happiness after talking about their problems:

> She felt she was part of it and had something in common with the others, even though she is usually not a 'joiner'.

> It made him feel important – like he was a leader in opening up.

> She thought she was the leader of the group members.

> Before meetings, he was high-spirited and excited to come. I [wife] tended to forget the meeting was coming more than he did – he never forgot. He looked forward to it and made his own transportation arrangements.

> She was reluctant to go at first. Then, eager from then on – she practically left me [husband] before getting to the meeting room.

He felt calm and upbeat after the meetings. He said beautiful and profound things to me [wife] at these times – he was very open emotionally.

Caregivers all thought their relatives' lives had changed as a result of the group; specifically, patients feeling more reassured, calmer, and more open about AD:

Recently, he talked with our houseguests about AD – this was unusual.

He feels less alone. He's accepted having the illness and his understanding of the illness increased with the group.

Caregivers felt the group helped the patients by 'normalizing' their experience, improving mood, and adding organisation to the patient's life. 'He felt safe to express his concerns and accepted by others. He realised he wasn't the only one, and wasn't even as bad off as he thought.'

She did talk about the group after it ended and up to 3 weeks later.

There's more verbal exchange between [my wife and I] now.

It gave him a purpose, and some structure.

It helped him identify the cause of his behaviour. He's a little more comfortable with the illness – had support while coming to terms with it.

None of the caregivers had any concerns about how patients responded, and all wanted their relatives to continue attending a group. Caregivers expressed appreciation for the patients' experience, and surprise and frustration that other services were not available locally. One caregiver regretted that this group experience had not been possible even sooner in the course of the illness.

Discussion

This study established that early stage dementia patients who had been given a diagnosis of AD had responses and concerns which they could express in interviews and in a support group. Comparison between treatment and control participants did not show statistically significant differences or changes over time in outcome measures. However, few existing assessment instruments are sensitive enough to make distinctions specific to mild dementia or the early stages of caregiving. Data from supplemental clinical interviews do suggest that patients and caregivers perceived multiple benefits from the intervention which may have affected their well being. The study describes some of the issues unique to the early stages of AD and demonstrates positive reactions to a particular service approach – suggesting that patient support groups are warranted, feasible and potentially therapeutic at this point in the disease course.

There are several limitations in this research. Study results apply only to those who met the inclusion criteria. Limited time and resources made it impossible to measure longer-range effects of the intervention. The pilot nature of the project necessitated a small sample size and scope. Furthermore, the occurrence of other events which created additional stresses in the lives of patients and caregivers (e.g. deaths of friends) made it difficult to isolate the impact of this intervention alone.

Replication can be undertaken to determine effectiveness through larger studies with longer-term follow up. Assessment instruments and outcome measures sensitive to the diversity of mild dementia patients and their caregivers in terms of specific impairments, acceptance of the illness and adjustments required might be developed and standardised. Further research paralleling service expansion is encouraged because it is obvious that early dementia patients have many issues to discuss when given the opportunity. Patients in this study were articulate, attentive, insightful and empathic in the group setting, and experienced great relief in talking with others who had similar problems. The need for and potential benefits of group support appear, then, to be analogous to those of caregivers and individuals with other common problems.

Group process issues are unique with the dementia population though, requiring facilitation techniques which accommodate patients' cognitive impairments and emotional reactions. Well-credentialled facilitators and careful screening of participants for mild memory loss, openness about diagnosis, and appropriate communication and social skills will maximise the chances that patients have the desire and ability to discuss their concerns about AD, and value the chance to do so.

Conclusion

> I'd like people to know – I've got a lot of life left…

Early dementia patients who seek information and support after receiving a diagnosis of AD currently have few places to turn for follow up. While AD patients have typically been dehumanised and regarded as unable to express their thoughts and emotions, subjects in this study described a sense of success and satisfaction from their participation. Professionals who assume there is little they can do for AD patients may not realise how much patients can accomplish for themselves. While it is challenging to be asked difficult, pointed questions about the illness, the window of time during which those who have it can act on information received is poignantly narrow. The longer they must wait for support groups to be available, the less likely it is that they will have the opportunity to experience one.

Thus there is a sense of urgency about the need for ongoing work in this area, and much that can and must be done. The intervention could be varied in length, size, and format; and modified to serve distinct subpopulations, such as patients of a specific age range, gender or culture. The development and evaluation of other programme components, such as concurrent or conjoint groups for caregivers, are extremely important. And finally, written materials which remind patients, families and professionals of the wellness (as well as the dysfunction) inherent in the early stages of dementia could serve an essential educational purpose.

Service providers across – and outside of – the country are increasingly aware of these unmet needs, and many are beginning implementation efforts. While support groups can't reverse or halt disease progression, they may help patients and their families understand the illness, address their concerns, and learn about other resources available to them. It is hoped that the findings presented here advocate strongly for initiation of public policy, continued research, and expanded programme development to create a 'new starting point' on the continuum of dementia care.

CHAPTER 16

Training and Younger People with Dementia

A Shared Learning Perspective

Alan Chapman

Introduction

The Health Advisory Service review report *Mental Health Services: Heading for Better Care* rightly identifies that 'Good training of staff is the core to any strategy to improve services' (HAS 1996, p.124). Particular obstacles exist in providing training in the dementia field, especially in relation to younger people with dementia. This is due to the diversity of causes, the range of specialisms involved and the pattern of service development. Identifying training needs in such a context can be challenging, both for service providers and those responsible for developing training at different levels. The problem is compounded by the ambivalent attitude that many practitioners have towards the idea of training when the issue is often seen as a lack of resources for professional and organisational support, and the practical considerations of taking time away from the workplace. Therefore there needs to be clarity about the objectives and outcome of training as well as careful consideration about the target audience and the training methods that are to be used.

A general aim of practice-based dementia care training is to improve knowledge and practice skills in relation to dementia. However, effective professional and service responses also depend on the ability of practitioners to work together in different settings and across service boundaries. A further important focus is therefore the promotion of interdisciplinary training.

The outcome of such training should be the sharing of knowledge, skills and expertise, greater insight and understanding of the needs of younger people with dementia resulting in more appropriate and responsive practice and services.

This chapter provides an overview of such issues and uses training initiatives at the Dementia Services Development Centre, Stirling, to illustrate particular approaches.

What is the meaning of training?

Training needs to be relevant to the needs of users and carers, the individual practitioner and the aims and objectives of the organisation. Ideally, it brings about both individual learning as well as organisational change in terms of better teamwork, communication, mutual understanding of roles, changes in work practice and service delivery.

At present, across many of the professional disciplines, there is a move away from predominantly didactic methods and the one-off training event to more planned opportunities for individuals to reflect upon their practice, using a problem-solving approach. This is based on the premise that the most effective adult learning is not one that gives immediate answers, but one which first discovers the relevant questions and problems. In other words, the emphasis is on experiential learning (Kolb 1984). Experiential learning proposes that adult learning comes about as a result of reflecting on experiences, forming ideas and testing out these ideas in practice which, in turn, leads on to new insights and experiences. In this model, learning is a continuous process grounded in the reality of experience and not necessarily dependent on new or specialist knowledge brought in by experts.

However, reflective practice and learning are skills which are not necessarily part of the routine activity of practitioners in direct care. Often due to pressures of work, staff teams may not take time to reflect on practice issues or problems until a crisis or critical incident occurs. Testing out, or putting into action, new learning requires opportunities for the learner to compare and identify how their practice has changed and improved. Carefully designed courses can provide the opportunity for individuals to take time to reflect upon their concerns, explore questions and find solutions. Real work problems are tackled rather than just acquiring new knowledge or theories in an abstract way. Therefore the training agenda should reflect the issues that concern the participants.

Margetson (1996), in discussing GP training, notes that problem-based learning makes explicit the initial understanding of the learner. The training course becomes an opportunity for the learner to recognise not only what they know, but what they need to know. As this approach uses concrete examples based on reflective practice new insights may be facilitated by the trainer. The learner, now seen as a partner in the process, takes responsibility for developing skills which integrate new learning with practice. In this approach the trainer is responsible for finding out from pretraining consultation, using peer discussion or a reference group approach, the particular matters that cause concern. For example, a recent workshop at the Dementia Services Development Centre explored the training needs of staff working with younger people (mainly in their 40s and 50s) who had not only a learning disability but also dementia. By focusing on real problems many common areas of concern were identified. Whilst some problems were directly related to gaps in knowledge, others had grown out of uncertainties about applying existing knowledge and expertise to new situations. Discussions about future training therefore needed to include opportunities for confidence building and developing support systems as well as more information about dementia care. Interestingly, many of the day-to-day problems had grown out of uncertainties in relation to interprofessional and interagency responsibilities and pointed to the need for an examination of policy and service development issues.

Shared learning

One of the greatest challenges for training professional staff is to cultivate an environment of shared learning where professional roles and their value bases are opened up for discussion and critical appraisal. Although the notion of a seamless service is agreed upon in theory, frequently in reality the 'problem' is often passed to another and there may be a tendency to blame other colleagues for not fulfilling their role when a situation has reached crisis point. Differences in attitudes and values of professionals are also exposed. Practitioners who promote 'ordinary life' principles working with younger people with dementia may reduce the emphasis on clinical issues.

Professional training often seems to close people off to shared values and problem-solving approaches. McMichael *et al.* (1995) identified how teachers and social workers prior to starting their respective professional courses held similar values and ideas about particular situations. After qualification they had moved further apart. Each group had adopted stereotypical attitudes towards the other.

A recent research project identified a disconnectedness between occupational therapy students' actual experience and ideal multidisciplinary participation in care planning. Hilton (1995) suggests: 'The paradoxical situation exists whereby an increasing awareness of the importance of the concept of teamwork to the well-being of clients prevails in a climate of fear of loss of individual professional boundaries and status.' If shared learning and teamwork skills are built in to professional courses, it should be easier for the particular collaborative approaches required in the field of dementia care, especially in younger onset dementia, to be carried through into practice.

Students from different disciplines could share the same core dementia curriculum as equals. Placements in work settings also become a means for the different disciplines to tackle the real problems and dilemmas that exist in providing support to younger people with dementia and their carers. Shared problem solving about a situation that involves the trainee GP, psychiatrist, nurse, social worker and occupational therapist creates effective learning but exposes each discipline to the knowledge, attitudes, skills, roles and duties of other professionals. The intended outcome is that after qualification each discipline is more likely to engage in effective team working, complementing each others' skills.

In reality good practice depends on each group of practitioners acknowledging their different value base and recognising the unique skills that each possesses. For example, in the learning disability field staff workers may find themselves involved with younger people with dementia and their relatives in having to come to terms with difficult information and decision making. This can lead to feelings of being overwhelmed if people do not feel competent in these new situations. Some staff will have worked with people with learning disability, but have little or no knowledge of dementia, a position summarised by Kerr: 'Others who have worked with older people will have knowledge and experience of working with people with dementia but know little about people with learning disabilities. Both groups have much to learn from each other.' (1997, p.1). Undoubtedly managers and supervisors are stakeholders in the training process. They have a role in creating an environment for learning which is 'bringing thinking and doing together' (Binney and Williams 1997, p.139).

A practical way of doing this is to use regular supervision time with individuals. An effort can be made to help the individual reflect upon particular situations. The outcome for the supervisor/manager, over time, becomes an increasing awareness of the individual's attitudes, skills and learning needs. For the practitioner there is an increasing recognition of their skills, knowledge and issues from practice which can lead to a clearer identification of work-related learning needs and personal development needs. Often these learning needs will be shared across the staff group.

The psychiatrist, neurologist, nurse, GP, social worker, occupational therapist, physiotherapist and speech and language therapist may all potentially be in contact with a younger person with dementia. Currently many of these disciplines in their professional training have relatively little academic or professional input on dementia, far less on younger onset dementia. Courses for the different disciplines need to include younger onset dementia so that students are aware of the existence of such conditions. This basic knowledge can then be the foundation for more specialist skills and knowledge. Knowledge is only one part of the answer. As important is the development of shared learning as part of professional training which can be a basis of fostering different attitudes to collaboration in practice.

The training curriculum

In planning and devising a training curriculum relevant to the needs of younger people with dementia, attention should be given to the underpinning principles which will inform the content. The training needs of the practitioners involved should also be identified. This may relate to general core knowledge and skills required for all but additionally, for those in specialist roles, reflect the need for specialist knowledge and provide them with opportunities to acquire new skills as well as refining current practice.

A fundamental principle of any training should be to promote the ethos of best practice. Those involved in developing and facilitating training courses need to be in touch with current developments in the field as well as relevant research and evaluation. Thus a dynamic relationship is required between commissioners, service providers and training organisations. The curriculum should also be informed by the users' and carers' views about their experiences of services and their ideas about appropriate outcomes.

Earlier chapters have identified user and care issues which need to be incorporated in training agendas. Communication skills are an essential foundation for much of this work. For practitioners such as the GP, community nurse, care manager or nurse in the acute hospital setting who are working with younger people with dementia there is a need to maintain and develop:

- observational skills which see the person behind the illness
- interpretive skills which recognise the uniqueness of each person and the importance of trying to understand why the person responds in a particular way
- communication skills which engage the person and promote self-determination and individuality both verbally and non-verbally
- planning and organisational skills which take account of users' and carers' views and use this knowledge to develop action plans which actively link the person to their past
- management skills which show awareness of others' roles, foster collaborative responses and appropriately link the person to the right level of support.

The training agenda also has to include a knowledge base which reflects the needs of practitioners. For instance, the lack of understanding about dementia by some practitioners and the unfamiliarity of other practitioners with the specialist knowledge base of an area such as learning disability. Consequently, training has to provide opportunities for practitioners to explore and develop:

- basic understanding of younger onset dementia and the implications for the individual and their families/carer/social network
- awareness of the different clinical conditions and pathways to care
- understanding of the care programme approach and individualised care
- planning/management
- multidisciplinary team working and ways of collaborating with other services
- an understanding of the role of specialist practitioners, identifying when it is appropriate to request specialist diagnosis and assessment and service responses.

If these are regarded as the core components for generalist practitioners, staff in specialist practice setting require to have specialist knowledge 'and maintain their general professional expertise' (HAS 1996, p.124). This will include understanding brain function and the pathology associated with younger onset dementia and specific conditions. For this group of staff, in-house training can be a means of sharing expertise, knowledge and creating problem-solving opportunities; such learning can be shared with wider specialist and generalist networks.

Regardless of service or agency setting such knowledge and skills are developed over time. This emphasises the need to have an ongoing process of training, which involves the learner in a dynamic learning relationship. The training agenda therefore is not restricted to the acquisition of facts and knowledge about the specific conditions within the younger onset field. It becomes a means to share expertise from real-life experiences across disciplines so that the networks of support for the individual and communication about service responses empower both the individual and the practitioner. Creative responses only occur when practitioners value each others' contributions and do not adopt insular attitudes. However this is not to the exclusion of using the findings from research and evidence based practice to inform a training programme. The lessons learned from such research can help practitioners focus on ways of developing more consistent and effective approaches to diagnosis, planning and service development. But how does training create a momentum for changing and improving practice and attitudes towards younger people with dementia?

Support staff

Many non-qualified staff both in hospitals and the community may be very involved in day-to-day support and work with younger people with dementia. Home care staff, nursing assistants and staff in day centres, group homes, residential and nursing homes frequently have little access to ongoing training opportunities. Such staff can benefit from a general understanding of dementia and its implications for those in the younger age groups. Evaluation of training courses at the Dementia Services Development Centre has shown that it is only when such staff become aware that difficult behaviour and losses in daily functioning are usually caused by the illness, and are beyond the control of the person with dementia, that there is a change in attitude. Training for support staff has to present best practice in relation to personal and social support and deal with the specific issues relating to particular conditions and settings.

Training in specific service settings

Younger people with dementia live in a range of settings including home, supported housing, nursing homes and hospital. Although they have the same basic needs as anyone else, they also have certain needs which require a more responsive and individualised approach. Staff in such settings as a special group home project for people with a learning disability, need to develop knowledge about the differences between the causes of dementia, acute confusional states, depression, physical illness and the effects of medication. People with a learning disability and dementia are also more likely to experience rapid changes in the progression of the illness and therefore require more frequent reviews and assessments of need. This means that practitioners have to develop assessment and intervention skills which focus on what the person can still do but give a level of support which compensates for increasing disability. More demands are made of practitioners in these situations and the focus of their communication and work should be 'maintaining people in their familiar and comforting environment for as long as possible' (Kerr 1997, p.73). Understanding the importance of a calm predictable environment is an important area of learning. This can be very different from the orientation of many projects for people with learning disabilities which are geared to 'ordinary living' approaches and has implications for how services are currently provided.

Training on specific topics

Specialist development and practice centres can bring managers and planners of services together to focus on issues such as design of living environments and offer consultancy to commissioning teams about service provision. They can also be proactive in bringing together specialist practitioners and non-specialists on particular topics such as challenging behaviour, HIV-related dementia and learning disability and dementia. The fact that issues such as challenging behaviour and maintaining daily living skills arise in the work of practitioners with older people with dementia as well as in work with younger people means that interest in developing sensitive responses transcends traditional professional boundaries and age-grouped services. Organising a training event on a particular topic will often reflect a cross-section of practitioners. Those attending can gain an appreciation of other professional views and attitudes but by engaging in shared learning exercises can begin to explore collaborative responses.

The Primary Care Training Initiative

This combined training and research project, set up in 1995 and funded by the British American Financial Services Community Trust and The

Robertson Trust, is attempting to act as a catalyst for GPs and community nurses to better address the needs of the person with dementia. The project objectives are based on research studies which show that GPs underdiagnose dementia in older people whilst district nurses, community psychiatric nurses and health visitors overidentify dementia, and provides one model of shared learning (O'Connor *et al.* 1988).

The project aims to:

- provide accurate and updated information on dementia, so as to encourage thorough early and comprehensive assessment
- assist practitioners in becoming more knowledgeable about non-medical services
- encourage the development of collaborative links with social services and other care agencies.

The underlying ethos of the project is that something can be done to maintain the quality of life for the person with dementia including younger people and that dementia is a topic necessitating ongoing learning by all members of the primary care team. A problem-solving case study approach is taken in the joint sessions. These are based on real case examples so that an exploration of critical incidents and care pathways can occur. All participants fill in a self-completion questionnaire, immediately prior to the training, after the training and four weeks on from the training. The purpose of this approach is to evaluate the impact of training on practice and to obtain information about participant's concerns about dementia. Findings then inform further training developments. Significantly, the aspects that cause concern to most participants often relate to lack of specific knowledge about dementia, assumptions about professional roles and, more crucially, an uncertainty about the role and provision of other community-based services. Although the training helps address these concerns it is very likely that for younger people with dementia, losses in ability, and functioning behaviour will be regarded as symptoms of the physical condition.

At present the project team see the need to introduce a session about providing support to younger people with dementia and their carers. The challenge of this training remains to engage all practitioners in reflective learning, prompt collaborative responses and develop evaluative frameworks to measure the effectiveness of interventions.

Involving carers in training with practitioners

A model adopted by the Kelty project (Adam, Chapman and Farnese 1992) involved carers and practitioners sharing the same training experience. The training aimed to provide information about resources and facilitate a greater understanding between health and social work practitioners and carers. Over a two-day course, timed to fit in with the carer's commitments at home, information about dementia was shared and discussions about professional perceptions and carers' concerns, continence management, welfare rights, challenging behaviour and communication were included as part of the programme.

Listening to carers and their concerns confronts assumptions by professional staff that they know best. The course also highlighted that carers looked for and expected a responsive service regardless of job title. If training is to work then it requires collaborative working on clear aims and objectives. For the carers attending this course, sharing the same training programme as local practitioners enabled an exchange of views and opinions and enhanced their confidence and self-esteem. Practitioners gained new insights and a different perspective on the stresses and demands of 24-hour caring.

Conclusion

This chapter has discussed the crucial role of training against a backdrop that younger people with dementia do not conveniently fit into current service provision. Professionals, support managers, staff and not least carers are stakeholders in an ongoing training process which acknowledges these real-world dilemmas and tensions. Creating learning opportunities which foster and empower staff potential whilst making an impact on practice is a real challenge. One solution is to focus on real problems so that practitioners from the various disciplines and settings share expertise, communicate and work together. Training therefore should not only be seen as acquiring knowledge but also as a dynamic means of staff working together to improve best practice in their work with younger people with dementia and those who care for them.

CHAPTER 17

Changing the Mind-Set
Developing an Agenda for Change
Sylvia Cox and John Keady

Introduction

Each author in this book has, in his or her own unique way, posed a set of challenges to stimulate an agenda for change for younger people with dementia, their families and support networks. We see this final chapter as complementary to each of these developments, providing an overview which challenges prevailing attitudes in society and, it must be said, within dementia care itself, by calling for a standpoint where planning, policy and services include younger people with dementia their families and support networks are considered as a matter of routine. The prevailing mind-set of dementia equating to older people resulting in older people's services must be actively challenged if any improvement is to be made. However, we also suggest that by highlighting the need for change in younger peoples' services we emphasise this need occurs in all age groups.

In order to integrate this agenda for change we have identified two distinct, but overlapping, themes, namely the need to:

1. Individualise care and service provision

2. Promote social integration not exclusion.

As a rule, diversity and equity in service provision are noble aims, but in practice remain competing areas for attention, making attempts at integration a complex (but not impossible) challenge for health and social care providers. As seen in Chapter 3 (Gregor McWalter and James Chalmers) younger people with dementia are often grouped alongside older people both in terms of assessment of need and service provision. This grouping is often rationalised on the basis that there is more knowledge and expertise about dementia in 'psychogeriatric' services. On the one hand, in terms of service provision and mode of service delivery, there may be a persuasive argument put forward to integrate services for younger people with dementia and those with learning disability, as the issues for carers are broadly similar (Nolan, Grant and Keady 1996). On the other hand, the ideal remains for a specialised multidisciplinary service for younger people with dementia encompassing early diagnosis and dedicated support services (for a working example see Ferran *et al.* 1996).

As Sylvia Cox discussed in Chapter 4, there still appears to be ambivalence, particularly on the part of policy makers, planners and practitioners in health and social care, to routinely including younger people with dementia on the service agenda. Why should this be? For a start, the range of need and (globally speaking) the relatively small numbers involved are obviously relevant. This was demonstrated quite starkly in a recent survey by the Alzheimer's Disease Society (ADS) with a number of their branches in the United Kingdom (UK) (ADS 1995). In this report it was found that only 20 per cent of health authorities had specific services for younger people with dementia, and most had no idea how many younger people with dementia existed in their catchment area. More worrying, the survey found that 94 per cent of the Society branches said that specialist residential care for younger people with dementia was not available in their locality.

The argument is not that younger people with dementia deserve better or more carefully developed services than older people, rather that they and their support networks (which includes employers, where relevant) have different, though intertwined, needs. These include:

- point in the life stage – life history and current roles, responsibilities and concerns
- changes to lifestyle – what people view as significant and meaningful in their lives
- retained mobility and physical strength
- the importance of dependent children, from infants to teenagers to grandchildren
- financial commitments and concerns
- genetic issues arising from a diagnosis
- family, friends and wider societal expectations about acceptable behaviour
- patterns of social contacts and networks

- attitudes to loss, death and on the meaning of their condition
- revisions in the expectations of ordinary everyday life, e.g. work, money, living arrangements, social and sexual relationships, independence and responsibility for others
- altered body image.

These factors are not exclusive to younger people, but taken as a whole will have a significant impact on the way that dementia is experienced by the person, their family and support networks. Here, we would suggest, the focus should be on the steps society needs to take to integrate younger people with dementia into mainstream and specialist service provision, and not simply rely on existing services to fit around the presenting circumstances.

In order to counteract social exclusion and marginalisation it is important to argue for positive steps to be taken to enable younger people with dementia to remain within their families and local communities with the appropriate dedicated level of support. There appears to be no reason why the kinds of service accomplishments set out by O'Brien (1987), which encompasses an inclusive philosophy, social participation, the promotion of competence and affording respect, should not be extended to all people with dementia and adapted to their individual needs and circumstances. Responding to each of these demands has implications for joint planning and priority setting, service objectives, patterns of working and staff attitudes and roles in the range of health, social care, housing and other community support services. These need to be underpinned by broader strategies involving increasing public awareness, health and social care education and promotion as well as a more collaborative and integrated approach to health and social care provision.

As we have seen during the book, a crucial strand in changing the mind-set is to acknowledge the disruption in the stages of the lifecycle and to campaign vigorously for early diagnosis and responsive support services. The balance of specialist and generalist services to respond to early diagnosis and support is thus very relevant. GPs are often seen as the generalist in primary health care and are mainly the first port of call in 'finding out what is wrong'. The skills of GPs in assessment and screening are crucial to case identification and, where available, to additional referral to other specialist support services, such as a memory clinic or neurologist. The complexities of pathways to services and user preference for a 'one-door' approach is understandable. However, at this time, the service is dependent upon the younger person with suspected dementia being able, and willing, to recognise they have a problem and to ask for help. Given the complex set of dynamics that are involved in this process, negotiating a successful path through this maze is not a simple matter as the uncertainty that exists at the onset of dementia only adds to the overall sense of confusion (see Chapter 10 by Diane Seddon and Chapter 12 by John Keady and Mike Nolan for further discussion).

In the UK, services for people with dementia have always hovered uneasily between services for mental health and those for older people. Until relatively recently, however, dementia was seen by social service agencies as primarily a health responsibility, but now the social care aspects are being highlighted much more vigorously (Social Services Inspectorate/Department of Health 1996). In reality social work has been providing for large numbers of the people with dementia through home care services, day and respite services and residential care, as well as commissioning and purchasing a range of mainstream and specialist care from the voluntary and independent sectors, including nursing home care. Housing providers, especially registered social landlords and housing associations, play an increasingly important role in partnership with social services and health authorities.

In the health service, consultants in old age psychiatry have had to compete with the acute sectors for their share of budgets and historically have tended to be more poorly staffed and resourced. Policies to reduce drastically the numbers of the longstay beds have further undermined morale and expertise without replacing it with, for example, an emphasis on complex care and treatment, intensive rehabilitation or enhancing skills in palliative and terminal care.

Much good work has been done and notable innovations and improvements in multidisciplinary practice and service have been achieved, but there still appear to be problems about local coordination and accessibility (Challis *et al.* 1997). The vision expressed in the recent UK government White Papers (DoH 1997; Scottish Office 1997c) is that closer partnerships between health and social care at more local levels will provide more effective services. It is vital that younger people with dementia are included in these local plans. Bearing this vision in mind, current policy guidance in the UK relevant to younger people with dementia can be synthesised as identifying that:

1. People should be supported in the community, preferably within their own home, rather than in institutions wherever possible.

2. Prevention of admission to hospital and long-term care through the pro-
    vision of locally based community living support systems should be pro-
    moted.

3. People with complex health and social care needs should have a
    long-term plan to ensure that their needs are assessed, monitored and re-
    viewed.

4. Sufficient funding should be available, by the reshaping and redistribu-
    tion of existing resources as well as additional funding through specific
    grants and programmes.

The development of care programmes, services and systems for younger people with dementia will need to be addressed across a range of client-specific
planning, for example mental health, learning disability, addiction and substance misuse, physical disability, HRBI, carer issues and such like. The kinds
of multidisciplinary and joint planning approaches will be influenced by a
range of factors, including attention to:

- values and principles
- strategic and more integrated planning between health, social work,
  housing and other agencies
- current resources and patterns of services
- estimates of unmet need
- public awareness and health promotion
- user and carer preferences
- care management, primary care and locality commissioning and development
- urban/rural issues
- social networks, levels of economic and social deprivation, ethnic and
  cultural diversity.

Effective planning involves gathering information about actual need at a
local level. However, the political, social and economic influences at strategic
level will also influence choices. In relation to the needs of younger people
with dementia it is important that the increasing emphasis on locality commissioning is informed by the need to collaborate across local boundaries to
provide appropriate levels of specialist service and expertise. Both specialist
and generalist services, such as primary care, are needed, but the coordination
between the two must be reconciled, the join continually monitored, evaluated and adjusted. Failure to address this issue will result in younger people

with dementia continuing to fall through the net of service provision and support.

Users and carers

Users and carers need to be more central in the planning process since this is the time that decisions are made about unmet need, priorities and patterns of service provision are discussed and shortfalls identified. This requires a continuing process of support and development via a range of support mechanisms including independent advocacy services, rights enshrined in service charters, standard-setting for user and carer involvement, funding user and carer organisations, information, advice and assistance. Within this book contributors have strenuously argued that younger people with dementia and their families need to be integrated into this process if improvement is to be made. As an ideal, this would include attention to:

Accessible information:

- locally based access and information on a 24-hour basis
- knowing where to go, information available on choice
- information about mainstream and specialist services as well as specific conditions.

Crisis response:

- available on 24-hour basis
- locally available
- a wider range of services including home-based supports
- somewhere for respite and security.

Long-term support:

- a broader range of housing and accommodation options
- help with accessing other mainstream community services
- participating in the decision-making process as long as possible
- a variety of home-based community living supports.

Local care coordination:

- one local access point for health and social work
- effective linkage between primary care and specialist services
- flexibility between services
- identification of one keyworker
- support for carers and families.

As we have seen in multidisciplinary working organisation and system arrangements are important but can only deliver if the professional and support staff involved have the knowledge, skills, positive attitudes and preparedness to learn and move across boundaries. The emphasis on education and training is reinforced in various chapters, however one of the most important features involved in changing the mind-set is to further emphasise the need to individualise care and support. In effect this involves ensuring that health, social care and other community support systems provide integrated and accessible pathways to multidisciplinary assessment and service provision. Effective and high-quality systems rely not only on professional expertise, knowledge and skill but on the dissemination and sharing of the practical application of such expertise with users and carers and non-specialist professionals and support staff.

The acceptance of shared values across service systems is more likely to result in person-centred services and developments which address the individualised needs of the younger person with dementia and those who care. Positive interagency and interprofessional working is required at planning, commissioning, system and practice levels if such developments are to become more generally available.

Person-centred planning emphasises the adult status of the person with dementia. It can be seen as a reaction against institutionalised and service-led approaches, an assertion of the centrality of the needs of the person with dementia and their well being. It suggests that solutions to problems must be located firmly in the specific needs of the person, as well as their significant others, and their specific social and personal situation, not stereotyped and packaged (Sanderson et al. 1997). Developments in the areas of employment, housing and palliative care point a way forward in putting into practice services and models of care which balance 'ordinary living' principles with the need for specialist knowledge and service support. On this former issue, for many younger people with dementia, the world of work is highly significant. For example, work may symbolise socialisation, income, regular routine, responsibilities, respect, self-esteem, meaningful activity and familiarity, and its sudden loss can be devastating. Withdrawing from the work environment and culture is recognised as a major life transition, and its removal can cause a profound sense of loss to the person's identity. Working with younger people with dementia involved in this transition requires both a sensitive and practical approach with, ideally, a more sheltered environment for its continuation.

At present there are a number of supported employment initiatives which can provide help for people with disability, with some schemes, such as the Kite Employment Services in Kent, including younger people with dementia. Naturally, the framework for a supportive environment for younger people with dementia incorporates a number of areas, and we would like to focus on three, namely: work schemes; housing preferences; palliative care.

Work schemes

We have divided these into a number of headings which we shall now address.

WORK SUPPORT

Using a case-management approach employers and colleagues can be helped to understand the person's needs and be advised about a range of intervention such as safety aspects, ways in which satisfactory work can still be completed, moving to a different type of work, retraining, early retirement courses, exploring best timing for retirement and pension prospects. Sometimes relationships may have deteriorated because people do not understand that the person has a particular condition, but people with dementia and those who care need help to share such information with others. Often work colleagues may be aware of changes in the person but do not know what to do about it.

ALTERNATIVE TYPES OF WORK

Such services need to be client-centred and involve getting to know the person and finding employment possibilities close to the person's home. Coaching and one-to-one work can help the person adjust to the new situation, often creating a positive corresponding effect in terms of the person's sense of dignity, relationship with others and continuity of past and present rather than an abrupt change to living at home all day which can lead to boredom, frustration and challenging behaviour.

MEANINGFUL LEISURE AND RECREATION

Paid work is closely related to other meaningful and worthwhile activity leisure and recreation. If work is interpreted in the widest sense then people will also respond to one-to-one support in accessing other community based activities. People can maintain or rediscover old skills and sustain them for varying periods of time. Depression is one of the most common conditions in the early stages, so enforced inactivity can be a major contributing factor, often exacerbating stress between family members.

EXPERIENCING A VALUED ROLE AND RESPONSIBILITIES

One of the most common occurrences is for younger people with dementia attending day centres for older people and seeing themselves as staff not attendees. In reality this is often the case since they often are physically fitter and can give help to the other more physically frail members – indeed staff often ask them to do so. They may also not be so advanced in terms of cognitive impairment and have more awareness of the situation. Such abilities, if carefully explored, supported and encouraged, might result in some work being found of a voluntary or leisure nature where appropriate adult status and recognition is given. A case manager may be able to find a range of ordinary activities in the community in which the person can participate with the support of relatives, friends and support staff, rather than escalating into formal day care before it is necessary. Further education courses, such as those in computer training for instance, have been able to offer appropriate courses to people with learning disabilities and it is not inconceivable that younger people with dementia could also be integrated into such provision.

Housing preferences

The continuity of past, present and future is important for any person with dementia, irrespective of age. Decisions about relocation should only be taken after every effort has been made to maintain independence in the community for as long as practicable, or desired. At the time of onset it is much more likely that the younger person with dementia will be living in the community as part of an integrated network which will involve a partner and/or close family members, together with other social responsibilities and routines. The home and surrounding environment, therefore, will have a significance not only for the younger person with dementia, but also for their family, friends, neighbours, schools and leisure pursuits. Obviously, planning ahead by making simple adaptations to the home is commonsense once the diagnosis is made and the individual and their family have come to terms with its meaning and impact upon their lives.

On the other hand, if a move is envisaged to supported housing or to be nearer other relatives, issues in housing needs becomes a priority. Features of the accommodation – such as ease of access, ground-floor setting, open layout, barrier-free design, available wiring for appropriate technology and its location relative to the availability of paid (formal) support staff – can make a significant difference to the quality of life. For the younger person with dementia considering a relocation may well involve an appraisal of available residential and/or nursing home accommodation as its provision for the younger person is, as we have seen, sparse to say the least.

Increasingly, it is accepted that people with dementia should have the right to their own tenancy, but will need varying degrees of support to ensure that they can maximise their remaining capacities:

1. Floating social and personal support provides flexible home support to people in their own homes. This is often combined with adaptations to the existing home environment or moving to purpose-built housing, often with dementia-friendly design features and new technology systems included. Good interagency working is required to ensure coordinated planning and care and there is usually a case manager and/or keyworker system.

2. Barrier-free homes of different sizes, supported by new technology and located in a mixed housing development, but close to a 24-hour staffed resource centre are another model. Staff are available to provide an appropriate level of care and support as and when needed; they may also provide individualised or small-group day activities or programmes. The availability of mixed housing types means that families can be accommodated without stigmatisation or marginalisation and families do not necessarily have to move again if the person with dementia has to be admitted to long-term care or dies.

3. There are a range of group housing models such as the one provided by the Dementia Care Initiative in Newcastle-Upon-Tyne in the UK (Svanberg, Stirling and Fairbairn 1997). Indeed, the approach varies considerably and depending on the tenure and funding system can be more like a shared tenancy, a grouping of individual houses or a small-scale group living unit where people live on a communal basis with paid staff available usually on a 24-hour basis. Ideally such developments are small – three to four people per house or groupings of six to eight houses. The principle of mixed housing is ideal since this creates more opportunities for normalisation and available housing for the person's family members or partner.

Naturally, it may not be possible to support everyone in a supported housing environment, but it should be considered an option for a much wider range of people.

Palliative care

Many young people with dementia will be cared for at home for much longer in their illness depending on the condition and the particular social network and support system. This is partly because there is more likelihood of them living with a partner/family, but also because it is less likely for other medical conditions to intervene as in the case of older people. For some people, admission to a nursing home or hospital will be unavoidable if there are difficulties about providing the right level of support at home, or there are specialised or complex medical or nursing needs.

Palliative care for the dying person with dementia has been a relatively neglected topic in relation to policy, planning, practice development and training. There are significant gaps in professional knowledge, skills and expertise, but there is an opportunity to cross-fertilise the fields of palliative and dementia care for the benefit of all concerned (Cox, Gilhooly and McLennan 1996). Issues identified and applicable for younger people with dementia include a need for:

- policy, planning and service coordination
- multiagency and interprofessional training
- resolving the issue of pain – impact on care and challenging behaviour
- models of palliative care in residential/nursing homes, hospital and home care.

In summary, palliative care is increasingly being provided at home, in the small housing type developments and group living as well as in residential and nursing care. Such care should be based on the principles of palliative care and dementia care, which are remarkably similar since they are based on a person-centred holistic and individualised approach.

Conclusion

Despite the steps outlined in this book, and elsewhere, to promote the value and specialised attention necessary for the coordination of care and service delivery to younger people with dementia, their families and support networks, it continues to be interesting to reflect upon why younger people with dementia remain such a neglected group, rarely being included at a strategic planning level in relation to hospital closures and resettlement projects, joint community care plans between health, social services, housing and voluntary agencies, in central government guidance or within individual service developments. It is apparent that at a systems level organisations do not appear to respond well to a diversity of need and small populations, and it is mainly left to campaigning organisations and user groups to draw attention to particular diseases, often by identifying a product champion to draw publicity. Partly, this is due to the need to raise money for research, development and support funds which, ironically, often has the effect of creating further barriers to cooperation and collaboration between groups. This creates a more central argument on needs and numbers with the planning and providing authorities. For example, competition for mental illness specific grant monies which exists between adult mental health services and those specialising in dementia is deleterious to the aim of quality services for both consumer groups and must be eradicated if the mind-set is to change and integration be achieved. This remains the responsibility of us all.

On a brighter note, the process of change has already started. Positive developments in relation to our understanding of the ways in which the biopsychosocial aspects of human beings interact and the detail of brain function along with continuing development of drug research hold out the prospect of improving quality of life and perhaps delaying, if not preventing, more disabling features. Therapeutic interventions highlighted by Bob Woods in Chapter 14 also point to a more positive way forward. Its continuation and development can be further promoted by:

- creating alliances across service and sector boundaries to ensure the maximisation of existing resources
- building on the strengths of the strong voluntary sector and user and carer organisations to campaign for more community awareness
- building on the strengths of professional networks across different areas of expertise
- embarking on a programme of public awareness and health and social care education and promotion
- involving and empowering users and their families and social networks in planning, service development, evaluation and research.

However, as we have intimated, it is perhaps to ourselves that we must turn to create the most meaningful change. We must encourage others and ourselves not to be fearful, to encourage inclusion and participation, to create community-based resources and to be creative and energetic in our search for positive solutions, especially by engaging with and involving younger people with dementia as well as their families and support networks. Only then, in our opinion, will the mind-set begin to change for the better.

The Contributors

Roseanne Cetnarskyj is an advisor at the Scottish Huntington's Association. Based in the Clinical Genetics Department at the Western General Hospital, Edinburgh, she provides a service for families affected by HD in Edinburgh and the Lothians.

Jim Chalmers is a Consultant in Public Health Medicine with the Information and Statistics Division of the National Health Service in Scotland. His current interests focus on information in primary, community and continuing care.

Alan Chapman is Training Officer at the Dementia Services Development Centre. He has written a number of publications in the dementia and training field.

Sally-Ann Cooper is Consultant in Learning Disabilities Psychiatry at St Mary's Hospital Rockingham Forrest NHS Trust. She has clinical responsibility for people with learning disabilities and dementia and has completed research studies on the subject.

Sylvia Cox is Planning Consultant at the Dementia Services Development Centre at the University of Stirling, Scotland. She is a qualified social worker and has previously worked as a practitioner and senior manager in community care. She is currently involved in consultancy, development and research in the field of dementia care.

Simon Crowe is Senior Lecturer in Neuropsychology at La Trobe University, Melbourne, Australia and is president of ARBIAS. He has a large number of publications in the field of neuropsychology.

Jane Gilliard is Director of Dementia Voice, the Dementia Services Development Centre for the South West of England. She has worked as a social worker and researcher in the field of dementia care.

Steve Jamieson is Lecturer in HIV and Sexual Health at the Bethlem and Maudsley NHS Trust in London. He has worked in the area of HIV/AIDS in hospital and in the community.

John Keady is Lecturer in Nursing at the School of Nursing and Midwifery at the University of Wales, Bangor. He previously worked as a community psychiatric nurse in dementia care team. He has a number of publications in the dementia field.

John Killick is a freelance writer and Writer-in-Residence for Westminster Health Care and the Dementia Services Development Centre at the University of Stirling. He has a number of publications and runs training courses in communication.

Jane McLennan is a Consultant in Old Age Psychiatry at the Royal Victoria Hospital, Edinburgh. She is also an Honorary Senior Lecturer at the University of Stirling.

Gregor McWalter is Senior Health Information Scientist with the Information and Statistics Division of the National Health Service in Scotland. He has been closely involved in developing needs assessment tools for people with dementia and relating this to strategic planning.

Mike Nolan is Professor of Gerontological Nursing and Director of Research at the School of Nursing and Midwifery at the University of Sheffield. He has a long history in developing research with family carers and in particular those caring for people with chronic illness.

Gretta Peachment is Consultant for Facilities and Planning at the Brightwater Care Group, Western Australia. She has extensive experience in design and facilities planning for people with dementia, including younger people, and has published in the field.

Mary Porteous is a Consultant and Senior Lecturer at the Department of Clinical Genetics at the Western General Hospital in Edinburgh. She has a particular interest in development and co-ordination of genetic services in the south east of Scotland.

Diane Seddon is a Research Officer at the Centre for Social Policy Research and Development at the University of Wales, Bangor. She has a long standing interest in issues to do with caregiving and employment, and is currently involved in an evaluative study on the Carer's Act.

Kirstie Woodburn is Specialist Registrar in Old Age Psychiatry at the Royal Edinburgh Hospital currently completing her M.D. in younger onset dementia.

Bob Woods is Professor of Clinical Psychology of the Elderly at the University of Wales, Bangor. He has a wide range of experience and a large number of publications in the dementia field.

Robyn Yale is an independent clinical social worker who practices in San Francisco, USA. She has extensive experience in group work with people with dementia and their carers and has researched the subject.

References

Adam, E., Chapman, A. and Farnase, R. (1992) *Carers and Professionals Together*. Stirling: Dementia Services Development Centre.

Aldridge, J. and Becker, S. (1993) *Children who Care – Inside the World of Young Carers*. Leicestershire: Loughborough University.

Alzheimer's Disease Society (1991) *Declaration of Rights For Younger People With Dementia and Their Carers* (leaflet). London: ADS.

Alzheimer's Disease Society (1992a) *The Younger Person with Dementia*. London: ADS.

Alzheimer's Disease Society (1992b) *Younger-onset Dementia (information pamphlet)*. London: ADS.

Alzheimer's Disease Society (1995) *Services for Younger People with Dementia: A Report by the Alzheimer's Disease Society*. London: ADS.

Alzheimer's Disease Society (1996) *Younger People with Dementia: A Review and a Strategy*. London: ADS.

Amar, K. and Wilcock, G. (1996) 'Vascular dementia'. *British Medical Journal 312*, 227–231.

American Psychiatric Association (1987) *Diagnostic and Statistical Manual of Mental Disorders*, 3rd edn – revised (DSM-III-R). Washington, DC: APA.

American Psychiatric Association (1994) *Diagnostic and Statistical Manual of Mental Disorders*, 4th edn – revised (DSM-IV-R). Washington, DC: APA.

Ames, D., Flicker, D. and Helme, R.D. (1992) 'A memory clinic at a geriatric hospital: Rationale, routine and results from first 100 patients.' *Medical Journal of Australia 156*, 9, 618–622.

Backman, L. (1992) 'Memory training and memory improvement in Alzheimer's disease: rules and exceptions.' *Acta Neurologia Scandinavica, Supplement 139*, 84–89.

Baker, R., Dowling, Z., Wareing, L.A., Dawson, J., and Assey, J. (1997) 'Snoezelen: its long-term and short-term effects on older people with dementia'. *British Journal of Occupational Therapy, 60*, 5, 213–218.

Baldwin, R.C. (1994) 'Acquired cognitive impairment in the presenium,' *Psychiatric Bulletin 18*, 463–465.

Ballard, C., Boyle, A., Bowler, C., and Lindesay, J. (1996) 'Anxiety disorders in dementia sufferers.' *International Journal of Geriatric Psychiatry 11*, 987–990.

Barber, R. (1997) 'A survey of services for younger people with dementia.' *International Journal of Geriatric Psychiatry 12*, 951–954.

Barnett, E. (1997) 'Collaboration and interdependence: care as a two-way street.' In M. Marshall (ed) *State of the Art in Dementia Care*. London: CPA.

Beresford, B. (1994) *Positively Parents: Caring for a Severely Disabled Child*. London: HMSO.

Berlyne, N. (1972) 'Confabulation.' *British Journal of Psychiatry 120*, 31–39.

Binney, G. and Williams, C. (1997) *Leaning into the Future. Changing the Way People Change Organisations*. London: Nicholas Brealey Publishing.

Bird, M., Alexopoulous, P. and Adamowicz, J. (1995) 'Success and failure in five case studies: use of cued recall to ameliorate behaviour problems in senile dementia.' *International Journal of Geriatric Psychiatry 10*, 305–311.

Bjømeby, S. (in press) 'The Besta flat in Tonsberg: using technology in houses for people with dementia.' *Proceedings Cognitive and Affective Disorders in the Elderly.* Publication forthcoming.

Bourgeois, M.S. (1990) 'Enhancing conversation skills in patients with Alzheimer's disease using a prosthetic memory aid.' *Journal of Applied Behavior Analysis 23*, 29–42.

Bowen, D.L., Lane, H.C. and Franci, A.S. (1986) 'Immunological abnormalities in AIDS.' *Progress in Allergy 37*, 207–223.

Bradshaw, J. (1972) 'The concept of social need.' *New Society 30*, 640–643.

Brooker, D.J.R., Snape, M., Johnson, E., Ward, D. and Payne, M. (1997) 'Single case evaluation of the effects of aromatherapy and massage on disturbed behaviour in severe dementia.' *British Journal of Clinical Psychology 36*, 2, 287–296.

Brownlie, J. (1991) *A Hidden Problem? Dementia Amongst Minority Ethnic Groups.* Stirling: Dementia Services Development Centre.

Burgio, L., Engel, B.T., McCormick, K., Hawkins, A. and Scheve, A. (1988) 'Behavioral treatment for urinary incontinence in elderly inpatients: initial attempts to modify prompting and toileting procedures'. *Behavior Therapy 19*, 345–57.

Burgio, L.D., Burgio, K.L., Engel, B.T. and Tice, L.M. (1986) 'Increasing distance and independence of ambulation in elderly nursing home residents.' *Journal of Applied Behavior Analysis 19*, 357–366.

Butterworth, R.F. (1995) 'The role of liver disease in alcohol-induced cognitive defects'. *Alcohol Health and Research World 19*, 122–129.

Cameron, K. and O'Neill, K.F. (1997) 'The CARD Project: co-ordination of assessment and resources in dementia.' *Scottish Medicine 17*, 1, 7–9.

Cameron, K., O'Neill, K.F. and Ferguson, J. (1998) 'Across the great divide.' *Journal of Dementia Care, 6*, 3, 11–12.

Camp, C.J., Foss, J.W., O'Hanlon, A.M. and Stevens, A.B. (1996) 'Memory interventions for persons with dementia.' *Applied Cognitive Psychology 10*, 193–210.

Caro, A.J. (1977) Huntington's Chorea: A Clinical Problem in East Anglia. PhD thesis, University of East Anglia.

Centre for Policy on Ageing (1990) *Community Life: A Code of Practice for Community Care.* London: Centre for Policy on Ageing.

Challis, D., von Abendorff, R., Brown, P. and Chesterman, J. (1997) 'Care management and dementia: an evaluation of the Lewisham Intensive Case Management Scheme.' In S. Hunter (ed.) *Dementia: Challenges and New Directions.* Research Highlights in Social Work. London: Jessica Kingsley Publishers.

Christie, A.B. and Wood, E.R.M. (1988) 'Age, clinical features and prognosis.' *International Journal of Geriatric Psychiatry 8*, 553–559.

Chui, H.C., Victoroff, J.I., Margolin, D., Jagust, W., Shankle, R. and Katzman, R. (1992) 'Criteria for the diagnosis of ischemic vascular dementia proposed by the State of California Alzheimer's Disease Diagnostic and Treatment Centers.' *Neurology 42*, 473–480.

Clarke, C.L. (1995) 'Care of elderly people suffering from dementia and their co-resident informal carers.' In B. Heyman (ed.) *Researching User Perspectives on Community Health Care.* London: Chapman and Hall.

Collinge, J., Owen, F., Poulter, M., Leach, M., Crow, T.J., Rossor, M.N., Hardie, J., Mullen, M.J., Janota, I. and Lantos, P.L. (1990) 'Prion dementia without characteristic pathology.' *Lancet 336*, 7–9.

Cooper, S.A. (1997a) 'High prevalence of dementia amongst people with learning disabilities not attributed to Down's syndrome.' *Psychological Medicine 27*, 609–616.

Cooper, S.A. (1997b) 'Psychiatric symptoms of dementia amongst people with learning disabilities'. *International Journal of Geriatric Psychiatry 12*, 662–666.

Cooper, S.A. (1997c) 'Deficient health and social services for elderly people with learning disabilities.' *Journal of Intellectual Disabilities Research 41*, 331–338.

Cox, S. (1991) *Pre-senile Dementia: an Issues Paper for Service Planners and Providers. Planning Report 1.* Stirling: Dementia Services Development Centre.

Cox, S.M. and McLennan, J.M. (1994) *A Guide to Early Onset Dementia.* Stirling: Dementia Services Development Centre.

Cox, S., Gilhooly, M. and McLennan, J. (1996) *Dying and Dementia.* Stirling: Dementia Services Development Centre.

Davies, S. (1996) 'Neuropsychological assessment of the older person.' In R.T. Woods (ed.) *Handbook of the Clinical Psychology of Ageing.* Chichester: Wiley.

Davis, R. (1989) *My Journey into Alzheimer's Disease.* Amersham: Scripture Press.

Delaney, N. and Rosenvinge, H. (1995) 'Presenile dementia: sufferers, carers and services.' *International Journal of Geriatric Psychiatry 10*, 597–601.

Dementia Relief Trust (1996) *The Care Must be There: Improving Services for People with Young Onset Dementia and Their Families.* London: Dementia Relief Trust.

Department of Health (1989) *Caring for People: Community Care in the Next Decade and Beyond* Cmd 849. London: HMSO.

Department of Health (1990) *The National Health Service and Community Care Act.* London: HMSO.

Department of Health (1993) *Monitoring and Development: Assessment Special Study. Joint SSI/NHSME Study of Assessment Pointers in Five Local Authority Areas.* London: Department of Health.

Department of Health (1997) *A Handbook on the Mental Health of Older People.* London: DoH.

Drake *et al.* (1995) 'Cognitive recovery with abstinence and its relationship to family history for alcoholism.' *Journal of Studies on Alcohol 56*, 104–109.

Duff, G. and Peach, E. (1994) *Mutual Support Groups.* Stirling: Dementia Services Development Centre.

Egan, G. (1990) *The Skilled Helper: A Systematic Approach to Effective Helping.* Belmont: Brooks/Cole Publishing.

El-Mallakh, R.S (1991) 'Mania and AIDS; clinical significance and theoretical considerations.' *International Journal of Psychiatry in Medicine 21*, 383–391.

Evandrou, M. (1995) 'Employment and care paid and unpaid work: the socio-economic position of informal carers in Britain.' In J. Phillips (ed.) *Working Carers.* Aldershot: Avebury.

Evans, E. (undated) *It's Me, Grandma! It's Me!* London: Alzheimer's Disease Society.

Evert, D.L. and Oscar-Berman, M. (1995) 'Alcohol-related brain impairments: an overview of how alcoholism may affect the workings of the brain.' *Alcohol Health and Research World 19*, 89–96.

Fearnley, K., McLennan, J. and Weaks, D. (1997) *The Right to Know? Sharing the Diagnosis of Dementia.* Edinburgh: Alzheimer Scotland – Action on Dementia.

Feil, N. (1993) *The Validation Breakthrough: Simple Techniques for Communicating with People with 'Alzheimer's Type Dementia'.* Baltimore, MD: Health Professions Press.

Ferran, J. and Wilson, K. (1997) 'Old Age Psychiatrist.' *Newsletter of the section of Old Age Psychiatry of the Royal College of Psychiatry*, No 6, March.

Ferran, J., Wilson, K., Doran, M., Ghadiali, E., Johnson, F., Cooper, P. and McCracken, C. (1996) 'The early onset dementias: a study of clinical characteristics and service use.' *International Journal of Geriatric Psychiatry 11*, 863–869.

Fleming, R.W. and Bowles, J.R. (1994) *Manual of the Revised Elderly Persons Disability Scale.* Australia: MacSearch, University of Western Australia.

Folstein, M.F., Folstein, S.E. and McHugh, P.R. (1975). '"Mini-Mental State": A practical method for grading the cognitive state of patients for the clinician.' *Journal Psychiatric Research 12,*189–198.

Freemon, F.R. (1976) 'Evaluation of Patients With Progressive Intellectual Deterioration' *Archives of Neurology 33,* 658-659.

Furst, M. and Sperlinger, D. (1992) *Hour to Hour, Day to Day: The Service Experiences of Carers of People with Pre-Senile Dementia in the London Borough of Sutton. Report.* Surrey: St Helier NHS Trust.

Garwick, A.W., Detzner, D. and Boss, P. (1994) 'Family perceptions of living with Alzheimer's disease.' *Family Process 33,* 3, 327–340.

Gelder, M., Gath, D., Mayou, R. and Cowan, P. (1996) *Oxford Textbook of Psychiatry.* Oxford: Oxford University Press.

Gibson, F. (1994) 'What can reminiscence contribute to people with dementia?' In J. Bornat (ed.) *Reminiscence Reviewed: Evaluations, Achievements, Perspectives.* Buckingham: Open University Press.

Gilliard, J. (1995) *The Long and Winding Road: A Young Person's Guide to Dementia.* Petersfield: Wrightson Biomedical Publishing.

Gilliard, J. (1996) 'Ripples of stress across the generations.' *Journal of Dementia Care 4,* 4, 16–17.

Glaser, B.G. (1978) *Theoretical Sensitivity: Advances in the Methodology of Grounded Theory.* Mill Valley, CA: Sociology Press.

Glaser, B.G. and Strauss, A.L. (1967) *The Discovery of Grounded Theory: Strategies for Qualitative Research.* Chicago: Aldine Publishing Co.

Goldsmith, M. (1996) *Hearing the Voice of People with Dementia: Opportunities and Obstacles.* London: Jessica Kingsley Publishers.

Gordon, D.S. and Spicker, P. (1997) 'Demography needs and planning: the challenge of a changing population.' In S. Hunter (ed.) *Dementia. Research Highlights.* London: Jessica Kingsley Publishers.

Grant, I. and Atkinson, J. (1987) 'Evidence of early central nervous system involvement in AIDS'. *Annals of Internal Medicine 107,* 828–836.

Green, G.R., Linsk, N.L. and Pinkston, E.M. (1986) 'Modification of verbal behavior of the mentally impaired elderly by their spouses.' *Journal of Applied Behavior Analysis 19,* 329–336.

Greene, J.G., Smith, R., Gardiner, M. and Timbury, G.C. (1982) 'Measuring behavioural disturbance of elderly demented patients in the community and its effects on relatives: a factor analytic study.' *Age and Ageing 11,* 121–126.

Gustafson, L. (1987) 'Frontal lobe dementia of the non-Alzheimer type: clinical picture and differential diagnosis.' *Archives of Gerontology Geriatrica 6,* 209–223.

Hachinski, V.C., Iliff, L.D., Zilhka, E., DuBoulay, G.H., McAllister, V.L., Marshall, J., Russell, R.W.R. and Symon, L. (1975) 'Cerebral Blood Flow in Dementia.' *Archives of Neurology 32,* 632–637.

Hamilton, M. (1960) 'A rating scale for depression.' *Journal of Neurology, Neurosurgery, and Psychiatry 23,* 56–62.

Hancock, L., Walsh, R., Henry, D.A., Redman, S. and Sanson-Fisher, R. (1992) 'Drug use in Australia: a community prevalence study.' *The Medical Journal of Australia 156,* 759–764.

Harper, C., Gold, J., Rodriguez, M., and Perdices, M. (1989) 'The prevalence of the Wernicke-Korsakoff syndrome in Sydney, Australia: a prospective necropsy study.' *Journal of Neurology, Neurosurgery, and Psychiatry 52*, 282–285

Harper, P.S. (1996) *Huntington's Disease*, 2nd edn. London: Saunders.

Haupt, M., Kurz, A. and Pollmann, S. (1992) 'Severity of symptoms and rate of progression in AD: a comparison of cases with early and late onset dementia.' *Dementia 3*, 21–24.

Hausman, C. (1992) 'Dynamic psychotherapy with elderly demented patients.' In G. Jones and B.M.L. Miesen (eds) *Care-giving in Dementia: Research and Applications*. London: Routledge.

Health Advisory Service (HAS) (1996) *Mental Health Services: Heading for Better Care*. London: HMSO.

Hilton, R. (1995) 'Fragmentation within interprofessional work. A result of isolationism in health care professional education programmes and the preparation of students to function only in the confines of their own discipline.' *Journal of Interprofessional Care 9*, 1, 33–40.

Hofman, A., Rocca, W.A., Brayne, C., Breteler, M.M.B., Clarke, M., Cooper, B., Copeland, J.R.M., Dartigues, J.F., Da Silva Droux, A., Hagnell, O., Heeren, T. J., Engedal, K., Jonker, C., Lindesay, J., Lobo, A., Mann, A.H., Molsa, P.K., Morgan, K., O'Connor, D.W., Sulkava, R., Kay, D.W.K. and Amaducci, L. (1991) 'The prevalence of dementia in Europe: a collaborative study of 1980–1990 findings.' *International Journal of Epidemiology 20*, 3, 736–748.

Holden, U.P. and Woods, R.T. (1995) *Positive Approaches to Dementia Care*, 3rd edn. Edinburgh: Churchill Livingstone.

Holland, A.J. and Oliver, C. (1995) 'Down's syndrome and the links with Alzheimer's disease'. *Journal of Neurology, Neurosurgery and Psychiatry 59*, 111–115.

Hulsegge, J. and Verheul, A. (1987) *Snoezelen: Another World*. London: Rompa.

Huntington's Society of Canada (1996) *Understanding Huntington's Disease*. Cambridge, Ontario: HSC.

Huxley, P., Hagan, T., Hennelly, R. and Hunt, J. (1990) *Effective Community Mental Health Services*. Aldershot: Avebury.

Jacobson, J.W., Sutton, M.S. and Janicki, M.P. (1985) 'Demography and characteristics of ageing and aged mentally retarded persons.' In M.P. Janicki and H.M. Wisniewski (eds) *Ageing and Developmental Disabilities, Issues and Approaches*. Baltimore, MD: Paul H. Brookes.

Jaffe, J.H. (1985) 'Drug addiction and drug abuse.' In A.G. Gilman, L.S. Goodman, T.W. Rall and F. Murad (eds) *Goodman and Gilman's Pharmacological Basis of Therapeutics*, 7th edn. New York: Macmillan.

Jagger, C. and Lindesay, J. (1993) 'The epidemiology of senile dementia.' In A. Burns (ed.) *Ageing and Dementia: A Methodological Approach*. London: Edward Arnold.

Johnson, M.L. (1986) 'The meaning of old age.' In S.J. Redfern (ed.) *Nursing Elderly People*. Edinburgh: Churchill Livingstone.

Josephsson, S., Backman, L., Borell, L., Bernspang, B., Nygard, L. and Ronnberg, L. (1993) 'Supporting everyday activities in dementia: an intervention study.' *International Journal of Geriatric Psychiatry 8*, 395–400.

Julien, R.M. (1995) *A Primer of Drug Action*, 7th edn. New York: W.H. Freeman and Co.

Keady, J. (1997) 'Maintaining involvement: a meta concept to describe the dynamics of dementia.' In M. Marshall (ed.) *The State of the Art in Dementia Care*. London: Centre for Policy on Ageing.

Keady, J. and Bender, M. (1998) 'Changing faces: the purpose and practice of assessing older adults with cognitive impairment.' *Health Care in Later Life: An International Research Journal, 3*, 2, 129–164.

Keady, J. and Gilliard, J. (in press) 'The early experience of dementia.' In T. Adams and C. Clarke (eds) *Dementia Care: Developing a Partnership in Practice.* London: Balliere Tindall.

Keady, J. and Nolan, M. (1993) 'Coping with Dementia: Understanding and Responding to the Needs of Informal Carers.' The Royal College of Nursing Research Conference, Glasgow, 4 April.

Keady, J. and Nolan, M.R. (1994) 'Younger-onset dementia: developing a longitudinal model as the basis for a research agenda and as a guide to interventions with sufferers and carers.' *Journal of Advanced Nursing 19,* 659–669

Keady, J. and Nolan, M. (1995a) IMMEL: assessing coping responses in the early stages of dementia.' *British Journal of Nursing 4,* 6, 309–314.

Keady, J. and Nolan, M. (1995b) IMMEL 2: working to augment coping responses in early dementia.' *British Journal of Nursing 4,* 7, 377–380.

Keady, J. and Nolan, M. (1996) 'Behavioural and Instrumental in Dementia (BISID): refocussing the assessment of caregiver need in dementia.' *Journal of Psychiatric and Mental Health Nursing 3,* 3, 163–172.

Keady, J. and Nolan, M. (1997) 'Raising the profile of young people with dementia.' *Mental Health Nursing 17,* 2, 7–10.

Keady, J., Nolan, M. and Gilliard, J. (1995) 'Listen to the voices of experience.' *Journal of Dementia Care 3,* 3, 12–14.

Kelly, H., Russell, E., Stewart, S. and McEwen, J. (1996) 'Needs assessment: taking stock.' *Health Bulletin 54,* 2, 115–118.

Kerr, D. (1997) *Down's Syndrome and Dementia.* Birmingham:Venture Press.

Killick, J. (1994) *Please Give Me Back My Personality! Writing and Dementia.* Stirling: Dementia Services Development Centre.

Killick, J. (1997) *'You are Words': Dementia Poems.* London: Hawker Publications.

King, E. (1993) *Safety in Numbers.* London: Cassell.

Kings Fund (1986) *Living Well into Old Age: Applying Principles of Good Practice to Services for People with Dementia.* London: Kings Fund.

Kitwood, T. (1997) *Dementia Reconsidered: The Person Comes First.* Buckingham: Open University Press.

Kitwood, T. and Bredin, K. (1992) 'Towards a theory of dementia care: personhood and well being.' *Ageing and Society 12,* 269–287.

Knight, B.G., Lutzky, S.M. and Macofsky-Urban, F. (1993) 'A meta-analytic review of interventions for caregiver distress: recommendations for future research.' *Gerontologist 33,* 2, 240–248.

Kokmen, E., Beard, C.M., Offord, K.P. and Kurland, L.T. (1989) 'Prevalence of medically diagnosed dementia in a defined United States population: Rochester Minnesota January 1 1975.' *Neurology 39,* 773–776.

Kolb, D. (1984) *Experiential Learning.* New Jersey: Prentice Hall.

Kopelman, M. (1995) 'The Korsakoff syndrome.' *British Journal of Psychiatry 166,* 154–173.

Kuhlman, G.J., Wilson, H.S., Hutchinson, S.A. and Wallhagen, M. (1991) 'Alzheimer's disease and family caregiving: critical synthesis of the literature and research agenda.' *Nursing Research 40,* 6, 331–337.

Lazarus, R.S. (1966) *Psychological Stress and the Coping Process.* New York: McGraw Hill.

Lazarus, R.S. and Folkman, S. (1984) *Stress Appraisal and Coping.* New York: Springer.

Lewis, J. and Meredith, B. (1988) *Daughters Who Care.* London: Routledge and Kegan Paul.

Linn, M.W., Sculthorpe, W.B., Evje, M., *et al.* (1969) 'A social dysfunction rating scale.' *Journal of Psychiatric Research 6,* 299–306.

Lishman, W.A. (1990) 'Alcohol and the brain.' *British Journal of Psychiatry 156,* 635–644.

Liston, E.H. (1979) 'The clinical phenomenology of presenile dementia: a critical review of the literature.' *The Journal of Nervous and Mental Disease 167*, 6, 329–336.

Lucca, U., Comelli, M., Tettamanti, M., Tiraboschi, P. and Spagnoli, A. (1993) 'Rate of progression and prognostic factors in Alzheimer's disease: a prospective study.' *Journal of the American Geriatric Society 41*, 45–49.

Lund, J. (1985) 'The prevalence of psychiatric morbidity in mentally retarded adults.' *Acta Psychiatrica Scandinavica 72*, 563–570.

Mackay, I.R. (1992) 'Dimensions and effects of alcohol abuse: a Victorian perspective and future directions.' *Victorian Health Promotion Foundation, Research Report Number 2.*

Maguire, C.P., Kirby, M., Coen, R., Coakley, D., Lawlor, B.A. and O'Neill, D. (1996) 'Family members' attitudes toward telling the patient with Alzheimer's disease their diagnosis.' *British Medical Journal 313*, 529–530.

Marder, K., Tang, M.K., Cote, L., Stern, Y. and Mayeux, R. (1995) 'The frequency and associated risk factors for dementia in patients with Parkinson's disease.' *Archives of Neurology 52*, 695–701.

Margetson, D. (1996) 'Beginning with the essentials: why problem based learning begins with problems.' *Education for Health 9*, 1, 61–69.

Marsden, C.D. and Harrison, M.J.G. (1972) 'Outcome of Investigation of Patients with Presenile Dementia.' *British Medical Journal 2*, 249–252.

Martin Matthews, A. and Campbell, L.D. (1995) 'Gender roles, employment and informal care.' In S. Arbert and J. Ginn (eds) *Connecting Gender and Ageing: Sociological Approaches to Gender Relations in Later Life.* Buckingham: Open University Press.

McArthur, J. and Hover, D.R. (1993) 'Dementia in AIDS patients; incidence and risk factors.' *Neurology 43*, 2245–2252.

McEwen, J., Russell, E. and Stewart, S. (1995) 'Needs assessment in Scotland: collaboration in public health.' *Public Health 109*, 179–185.

McGonigal, G., Thomas, B.M., McQuade, C.A., Starr, J.M., MacLennan, W.J. and Whalley, L.J. (1993) 'Epidemiology of Alzheimer's presenile dementia in Scotland 1974–88.' *British Medical Journal 306*, 680–683.

McGowin, D.F. (1993) *Living in the Labyrinth: A Personal Journey Through the Maze of Alzheimer's.* San Francisco: Elder Books.

McKeith, I.G., Fairbairn, A.F., Perry, R.H. and Thomson, P. (1994) 'The clinical diagnosis and misdiagnosis of senile dementia of Lewy Body type.' *British Journal of Psychiatry 165*, 324–332.

McKhann, G., Drachman, D., Folstein, M., Katzman, R., Price, D. and Stadlan, E.M. (1984) 'Clinical diagnosis of Alzheimer's disease: report of the NINCDS-ADRDA Work Group under the auspices of Department of Health and Human Services Task Force on Alzheimer's Disease.' *Neurology 34*, 939–943.

McLaughlin, E. and Ritchie, J. (1994) 'Legacies of caring: the experiences and circumstances of ex-carers.' *Health and Social Care 2*, 241–253.

McMichael, P., Grice, C., Garwood, F. and McDowall, S. (1995) *Peacemaking Among the Tribes,* Stirling: Dementia Services Development Centre.

McMurdo, M.E.I., Grant, D.G., Gilchrist, J., Findlay, D. and McLennan, J.M. (1993) 'The Dundee Memory Clinic: the first 100 patients.' *Health Bulletin 51*, 4, 203–207.

McWalter, G. (1997) 'What do we mean when we talk about assessment?' In M. Marshall (ed.) *State of the Art in Dementia Care.* London: Centre for Policy on Ageing.

McWalter, G., Toner, H., Corser, A., Eastwood, J., Marshall, M. and Turvey, T. (1994) 'Needs and needs assessment: their components and definitions with reference to dementia.' *Health and Social Care in the Community 2*, 4, 213–270.

McWalter, G., Tones, H., McWalker, A., Eastwood, J., Marshall, M. and Turvey, T. (1998) 'A community needs assessment: The Care Needs Assessment Pack for Dementia (CareNAPD) – its development, reliability and validity.' *International Journal of Geriatric Psychiatry 13,* 16–22.

Miesen, B.M.L. and Jones, G.M.M. (1997) *Care-giving in Dementia: Research and Applications,* Vol. 2. London: Routledge.

Miller, E. and Morris, R. (1993) *The Psychology of Dementia.* Chichester: Wiley.

Mills, M.A. (1997) 'Narrative identity and dementia: a study of emotion and narrative in older people with dementia.' *Ageing and Society 17,* 673–698.

Ministerial Task Force on Dementia Services in Victoria (1997) *Dementia Care in Victoria: Building a Pathway to Excellence.* Melbourne: Human Services Communications Unit.

Moffat, N., Barker, P. Pinkney, L., Garside, M. and Freeman, C. (1993) *Snozelen: An Experience for People with Dementia.* Chesterfield: Rompa.

Molsa, P.K., Marttila, R.I. and Rinne, U.K. (1982) 'Epidemiology of dementia in a Finnish population.' *ActaNeurologica Scandanavica 65,* 541–552.

Morris, R.G., and McKiernan, F. (1994) 'Neuropsychological investigation of dementia.' In A. Burns and R. Levy (eds) *Dementia.* London: Chapman & Hall.

Moss, S. and Patel, P. (1993) 'The prevalence of mental illness in people with intellectual disability over 50 years of age, and the diagnostic importance of information from carers.' *The Irish Journal of Psychology 14,* 110–129.

Moss, S., Patel, P. (1995) 'Psychiatric symptoms associated with dementia in older people with learning disability.' *British Journal of Psychiatry 167,* 663–7.

Mulligan, T.E. (1994) Service and Policy Issues for Younger Age Group Dementia Sufferers: A Nursing Perspective. MSc Dissertation, School of Nursing Studies, University of Bradford.

Naegele, G. and Reichert, M. (1995) 'Eldercare and the workplace: a new challenge for all social partners in Germany.' In J. Phillips (ed.) *Working Carers.* Aldershot: Avebury.

National Health and Medical Research Council (1987) *Is There a Safe Level of Daily Consumption of Alcohol for Men and Women? Recommendations Regarding Responsible Drinking Behaviour.* Canberra: Australian Government Printing Office.

Navia, B.A. and Jordan, B. (1986) 'The AIDS dementia complex. I Clinical Features.' *Annals of Neurology 19,* 517–521.

Navia B.A., Cebo, E.S., Petito, C.K. and Price, R.W. (1986) 'The AIDS dementia complex. II Neuropathology.' *Annals of Neurology 19,* 525–535.

Navia, B.A. and Price, R.W. (1987) 'The acquired immunodeficiency syndrome dementia complex as the presenting or sole manifestation of human immunodeficiency virus infection.' *Archives of Neurology 44,* 65–69.

Neal, M., Chapman, N., Ingersoll-Dayton, B. and Emlen, A. (1993) *Balancing Work and Caregiving for Children, Adults and Elders.* New York: Sage.

Netten, A. (1993) *A Positive Environment? Physical and Social Influences on People with Senile Dementia in Residential Care.* Aldershot: Ashgate.

Newens, A.J., Forster, D.P. and Kay, D.W.K. (1995) 'Dependency and community care in presenile Alzheimer's disease.' *British Journal of Psychiatry 166,* 777–782.

Newens, A.J., Forster, D.P., Kay, D.W.K., Kirkup, W., Bates, D. and Edwardson, J. (1993) 'Clinically diagnosed presenile dementia of the Alzheimer type in the Northern Health Region: ascertainment prevalence incidence and survival.' *Psychological Medicine 23,* 631–644.

NHS Health Advisory Service (1996) *Mental Health Services: Heading for Better Care.* London: The NHS Health Advisory Service.

Nocon, A. and Qureshi, H. (1996) *Outcomes of Community Care for Users and Carers: A Social Services Perspective.* Buckingham: Open University Press.

Nolan, M. and Caldock, K. (1995) 'Assessment: identifying the barriers to good practice.' *Health and Social Care in the Community 4,* 2, 77–85.

Nolan, M. and Grant, G. (1992) *Regular Respite: An Evaluation Of A Hospital Rota Bed Scheme For Elderly People,* Age Concern Institute of Gerontology Research Paper No. 6. London: ACE Books.

Nolan, M., Grant, G., Caldock, K. and Keady, J. (1994) *A Framework for Assessing the Needs of Family Carers: A Multi-disciplinary Guide.* Stoke-on-Trent: BASE Publications.

Nolan, M., Grant, G. and Keady, J. (1996) *Understanding Family Care: A Multidimensional Model of Caring and Coping.* Buckingham: Open University Press.

Nolan, M., Keady, J. and Grant, G. (1995) 'Developing a typology of family care: implications for nurses and other service providers.' *Journal of Advanced Nursing 21,* 256–265.

Nott, P.N. and Fleminger, J.J. (1975) 'Presenile dementia: the difficulties of early diagnosis.' *Acta Psychiatrica Scandanavica 51,* 210–217.

O'Brien, J. (1987) 'A guide to personal futures planning.' In G.T. Bellamy and B. Wilcox (eds) *A Comprehensive Guide to the Activities Catalogue: An Alternative Curriculum for Youth and Adults with Severe Disabilities.* Baltimore, MD: Paul H. Brookes.

O'Brien, J., Pearpoint, J. and Forrest, M. (1993) *PATH: Planning Alternative Tomorrow's with Hope – A Workbook for Planning Possible Positive Futures.* Toronto: Inclusion Press.

O'Connor, D.W., Pollitt, P.A., Hyde, J.B. *et al.* (1988) 'Do general practitioners miss dementia in elderly patients?' *British Medical Journal 297,* 1107–1110.

Oliver, C. and Holland, A.J. (1986) 'Down's syndrome and Alzheimer's disease: a review.' *Psychological Medicine 16,* 307–322.

Øvretveit, J. (1993) *Coordinating Community Care: Multidisciplinary Teams and Care Management.* Buckingham: Open University Press.

Parker, G. (1993) *With This Body: Caring and Disability in Marriage.* Buckingham: Open University Press.

Patmore, C. and Weaver, T. (1991) *Community Mental Health Teams: Lessons for Planners and Managers.* London: Good Practice in Mental Health.

Pattie, A.H. and Gillcard, C.J. (1979) *Manual of the Clifton Assessment Procedures for the Elderly.* Sevenoaks: Hodder and Stoughton.

Peachment, G. (in press) 'Designing the built environment for people with dementia, Parkinson's and Huntington's disease.' *Proceedings of the IAHSA Conference, Trends in Care and Housing for the Ageing.* Barcelona: Publication forthcoming.

Pearlin, L.I., Mullan, J.T., Semple, S.J. and Skaff, M.M. (1990) 'Caregiving and the stress process: an overview of concepts and their measures.' *The Gerontologist 30,* 5, 583–591.

Peck, D.F. and Shapiro, C.M. (1990) 'Guidelines for the construction selection and interpretation of measurement devices.' In D.F. Peck and C.M. Shapiro (eds) *Measuring Human Problems.* Chichester: Wiley.

Perry, R.H., Irving, D., Blessed, G., Fairbairn, A. and Perry, E.K. (1990) 'Senile dementia of the Lewy Body type.' *Journal of Neurological Science 95,* 119–139.

Phillips, J. (1995) 'Introduction.' In J. Phillips (ed.) *Working Carers.* Aldershot: Avebury.

Philp, I., McKee, K.J., Meldrum, P., Ballinger, B.R., Gilhooly, M.L.M., Gordon, D.S., Mutch, W.J. and Whittick, J.E. (1995) 'Community care for demented and non-demented elderly people: a comparison study of financial burden service use and unmet needs in family supporters.' *British Medical Journal 310,* 1503–1506.

Pinkston, E.M., and Linsk, N.L. (1984) *Care of the Elderly – A Family Approach.* New York: Pergamon.

Prasher, V.P. (1995) 'Age specific prevalence, thyroid dysfunction and depressive symptomatology in adults with Down syndrome and dementia.' *International Journal of Geriatric Psychiatry 10*, 25–31.

Prasher, V.P. and Filer, A. (1995) 'Behavioural disturbance in people with Down's syndrome and dementia.' *Journal of Intellectual Disability Research 39*, 432–436.

Price, R.W. and Brew B.J. (1988) 'AIDS commentary: the AIDS dementia complex.' *Journal of Infectious Diseases 158*, 1079–1083.

Quarrell, A.W.J., Tyler, A., Jones, M.P., Nordin, M. and Harper, P.S. (1988) 'Population studies of Huntington's disease in Wales.' *Clinical Genetics 33*, 189–195.

Quinn, C. (1996) *The Care Must Be There: Improving Services for People with Young Onset Dementia and Their Families.* London: The Dementia Relief Trust.

Reifler, B.V. and Larson, E. (1990) 'Excess disability in dementia of the Alzheimer's type.' In E. Light and B.D. Lebowitz (eds) *Alzheimer's Disease: Treatment and Family Stress.* New York: Hemisphere.

Reisberg, B., Ferris, S.H., de Leon, M.J. and Crook, T. (1982) 'The global deterioration scale for assessment of primary dementia.' *American Journal of Psychiatry 139*, 1136–1139.

Rice, K. and Warner, N. (1994) 'Breaking the bad news: what do psychiatrists tell patients with dementia about their illness?' *International Journal of Geriatric Psychiatry 9*, 467–471.

Rogers, S.L., Farlow, M.R., Doody, R.S., Mohs, R. and Friedhoff, L.T. (1998) 'A 24 week double blind placebo-controlled trial of donepezil in patients with Alzheimer's disease.' *Neurology 50*, 136-145.

Rolland, J.S. (1988) 'A conceptual model of chronic and life threatening illness and its impact on families.' In C.C. Chiman, E.W. Nunnally and F.M. Cox (eds) *Chronic Illness and Disabilities.* Beverly Hills, CA: Sage.

Roman, G.C., Tatemichi, T.K., Erkinjuntii, T., Cummings, J.L., Masdeu, J.C., Garcia, J.H., Amaducci, L., Orgogozo, J.-M., Brun, A., Hofman, A., Moody, D.M., O'Brien, M.D., Yamaguchi, T., Grafman, J., Drayer, B.P., Bennett, D.A., Fisher, M., Ogata, J., Kokmen, E., Bermejo, F., Wolf, P.A., Gorelick, P.B., Bick, K.L., Pajeau, A.K., Bell, M.A., DeCarli, C., Culebras, A., Korczyn, A.D., Bogousslavsky, J., Hartmann, A. and Scheinberg, P. (1993) 'Vascular dementia: diagnostic criteria for research studies, Report of the NINDS-AIREN International Workshop.' *Neurology 43*, 250–260.

Ron, M.A., Toone, B.K., Garralda, M.E. and Lishman, W.A. (1979) 'Diagnostic accuracy in presenile dementia.' *British Journal of Psychiatry 134*, 161–168.

Rossor, M.N. (1996) 'BSE and human disease.' *Journal of the Royal College of Physicians 30*, 6, 494–495.

Royal College of Psychiatrists (1989) *HIV and Mental Health Review.* London: HMSO.

Rutter, M., Graham, P. and Yule, W. (1970) *A Neuropsychiatric Study in Childhood.* London: Heinemann.

Rutter, M., Tizard, J. and Whitmore, K. (1970) *Education, Health and Behaviour.* London: Longman.

Sanderson, H., Kennedy, J., Ritchie, P. and Goodwin, G. (1997) *People, Plans and Possibilities: Exploring Person Centred Planning.* Edinburgh: Scottish Human Services.

Scharlach, A.E. (1989) 'A comparison of employed caregivers of cognitively impaired and physically impaired elderly persons.' *Research on Aging 11*, 225–243.

Schnelle, J.F., Newman, D., White, M., Abbey, J., Wallston, K.A., Fogarty, T. and Ory, M.G. (1993) 'Maintaining continence in nursing home residents through the application of industrial quality control.' *Gerontologist 33*, 114–121.

Schoenberg, B.S., Anderson, D.W. and Haerer, A.F. (1985) 'Severe dementia prevalence and clinical features in a biracial US population.' *Archives of Neurology 42*, 740–743.

Scottish Huntington's Association (1996) *What is Huntington's Disease?* Eldeslie: SHA.

Scottish Needs Assessment Programme (SNAP) (1997) *Dementia*. Glasgow: Scottish Forum for Public Health Medicine.

Scottish Office (1997a) *A Framework for Mental Health Services in Scotland*. Edinburgh: The Scottish Office.

Scottish Office (1997b) *Scottish Needs Assessment Programme*. Glasgow: Scottish Forum for Public Health Medicine.

Scottish Office DoH (1997c) *Designed to Care: Reviewing the National Health Service in Scotland*. Edinburgh: Scottish Office.

Simpson, S. and Johnston, A.W. (1989) 'The prevalence and patterns of care in Huntington's chorea in Grampian.' *British Journal of Psychiatry 155*, 799–804.

Sinason, V. (1992) 'The man who was losing his brain.' In V. Sinason (ed.) *Mental Handicap and the Human Condition: New Approaches from the Tavistock*. London: Free Association Books.

Smale, G., Tuson, G., Biehal, N. and Marsh, P. (1993) *Empowerment Assessment Care Management and the Skilled Worker*. London: HMSO.

Smith, J.S. and Kiloh, L.G. (1981) 'The investigation of dementia: results in 200 consecutive admissions.' *Lancet I*, 824–827.

Social Services Inspectorate/Department of Health (1996) *Assessing Older People with Dementia in the Community: Practice Issues for Social and Health Services*. Wetherby: HMSO.

Social Services Inspectorate/Social Work Services Group (1991a) *Care Management and Assessment: Practitioners Guide*. London: HMSO.

Social Services Inspectorate/Social Work Services Group (1991b) *Care Management and Assessment: Managers Guide*. London: HMSO.

Social Work Services Inspectorate for Scotland (1996) *Population Needs Assessment in Community Care: A Handbook for Planners and Practitioners*. Edinburgh: HMSO.

Spaull, D., Leach, C. and Frampton, I. (1998) 'An evaluation of the effects of sensory stimulation with people who have dementia.' *Behavioural and Cognitive Psychotherapy 26*, 77–86.

Sperlinger, D. and Furst, M. (1994) 'The service experiences of people with pre-senile dementia: a study of carers in one London borough.' *International Journal of Geriatric Psychiatry 9*, 47–50.

Stevens, A. and Raftery, J. (1994) 'The epidemiologically based needs assessment reviews – introduction.' In A. Stevens and J. Raftery (eds) *Health Care Needs Assessment*. Oxford: Radcliffe Medical Press.

Stewart R. (1979) 'The nature of needs assessment in community mental health.' *Community Mental Health Journal 15*, 4, 287–295.

Stokes, G. (1996) 'Challenging behaviour in dementia: a psychological approach.' In R.T. Woods (ed.) *Handbook of the Clinical Psychology of Ageing*. Chichester: Wiley.

Stokes, G. and Goudie, F. (eds.) (1990) *Working with Dementia*. Bicester: Winslow Press.

Sulkava, R., Wikstrom, J., Aromaa, A., Raitasalo, R., Lehtinen, V., Lahtela, K. and Palo, J. (1985) 'Prevalence of severe dementia in Finland.' *Neurology 35*, 1025–1029.

Sutton, L.J. and Cheston, R. (1997) 'Re-writing the story of dementia: a narrative approach to psychotherapy with people with dementia.' In M. Marshall (ed.) *State of the Art in Dementia Care*. London: CPA.

Svanberg, R., Stirling, E. and Fairbairn, A. (1997) 'The process of case management with people with dementia.' *Health and Social Care in the Community 5*, 2, 134–139.

Taylor, P. (1987) 'A living bereavement.' *Nursing Times 83*, 30, 27–30.

Teri, L. and Gallagher-Thompson, D. (1991) 'Cognitive-behavioural interventions for treatment of depression in Alzheimer's disease.' *Gerontologist 31*, 413–416.

Thayer, R. (1973) 'Measuring need in the social services.' *Social and Economic Administration 7*, 91–105.

Thompson, L.W., Wagner, B., Zeiss, A. and Gallagher, D. (1990) 'Cognitive/behavioural therapy with early stage Alzheimer's patients: an exploratory view of the utility of this approach.' In E. Light and B.D. Lebowitz (eds) *Alzheimer's Disease: Treatment and Family Stress*. New York: Hemisphere.

Thomson, A.D., Pratt, O.E., Jeyasingham, M. and Shaw, G.K. (1988) 'Alcohol and brain damage.' *Human Toxicology 7*, 455–463.

Tibbs, M.A. (1995) 'Steering a course over troubled waters.' *Journal of Dementia Care 3*, 5, 14–16.

Tindall, L. and Manthorpe, J. (1997) 'Early onset dementia: a case of ill-timing?' *Journal of Mental Health 6*, 3, 237–249.

Treves, T., Korczyn, A.D., Zilber, N., Kahana, E., Leibowitz ,Y., Alter, M. and Schoenberg, B.S. (1986) 'Presenile dementia in Israel.' *Archives of Neurology 43*, 26–29.

Tuck, R. (1992) 'Alcohol and the brain.' *The Medical Journal of Australia 156*, 749–750.

Twigg, J. and Atkin, K. (1994) *Carers Perceived: Policy and Practice in Informal Care*. Buckingham: Open University Press.

Verhey, F.R., Jolles, J., Ponds, R.W., Rozendaal, N., Plugge, C.A., de Vet, R.C., Vreeling, F.W. and Van der Lugt, P.J. (1993) 'Diagnosing dementia: a comparison between a monodisciplinary and a multidisciplinary approach.' *Journal of Neuropsychiatry and Clinical Neuroscience 51*, 78–85.

Victor, M., Adams, R.M. and Collins, G.H. (1989) *The Wernicke- Korsakoff Syndrome*, 2nd edn. Philadelphia: F.A. Davies.

Victoratos, G.C., Lenman, J.A.R. and Herzberg, L. (1977) 'Neurological investigation of dementia.' *British Journal of Psychiatry 130*, 131–133.

Vitaliano, P.P., Young, H.M. and Russo, J. (1991) 'Burden: a review of measures used among caregivers of individuals with dementia.' *Gerontologist 31*, 1, 67–75.

Wagland, J. and Peachment, G. (1996) *Chairs: Guidelines for the Purchase of Lounge, Dining and Occasional Seating for Elderly Long-Term Residents*. Stirling: Dementia Services Development Centre.

Walsh, K.W. (1994) *Neuropsychology: A Clinical Approach*, 3rd edn. Edinburgh: Churchill Livingstone.

Walton, J. and Roques, P. (1994) 'Robbed of their future.' *Journal of Dementia Care 2*, 4, 20–22.

Welden, S. and Yesavage, J.A. (1982) 'Behavioral improvement with relaxation training in senile dementia.' *Clinical Gerontologist 1*, 45–49.

Wilcox, J., Jones, B. and Alldrick, D. (1995) 'Identifying the support needs of people with dementia and older people with mental illness on a joint community team: a preliminary report.' *Journal of Mental Health 4*, 157–163.

Will, R.G., Ironside, J.W., Zeidler, M. *et al.* (1996) 'A new variant of Creutzfeld-Jacob disease in the UK.' *Lancet 347*, 921–925.

Williams A. (1989) *Creating a Health Care Market: Ideology, Efficacy, Ethics and Clinical Freedom.* (NHS white paper occasional paper University of York.) York: York Centre for Health Economics.

Williams, D.D.R. (1995) 'Services for younger sufferers of Alzheimer's Disease.' *British Journal of Psychiatry 166*, 699–700.

Williams, O., Keady, J. and Nolan, M.R. (1995) 'Younger-onset Alzheimer's disease: learning from the experience of one spouse carer.' *Journal of Clinical Nursing 4*, 1, 31–36.

Wilson, H.S. (1989a) 'Family caregivers: the experience of Alzheimer's disease.' *Applied Nursing Research 2*, 1, 40–45.

Wilson, H.S. (1989b) 'Family caregiving for a relative with Alzheimer's dementia: coping with negative choices.' *Nursing Research 38*, 2, 94–98.

Woods, B. (1995) 'Dementia care: progress and prospects.' *Journal of Mental Health 4*, 2, 115–124.

Woods, R.T. (1996) 'Psychological "therapies" in dementia.' In R.T. Woods (ed.) *Handbook of the Clinical Psychology of Ageing*. Chichester: Wiley.

Woods, R.T. and Bird, M. (1998) 'Non-pharmacological approaches to treatment.' In G. Wilcock, K. Rockwood and R. Bucks (eds) *Diagnosis and Management of Dementia: A Manual for Memory Disorders Teams*. Oxford: Oxford University Press.

Woods, R.T. and Roth, A. (1996) 'Effectiveness of psychological interventions with older people.' In A. Roth and P. Fonagy (eds.) *What Works for Whom? A Critical Review of Psychotherapy Research*. New York: Guilford Press.

World Health Organization (1990) *Report of the Second Consultation on the Neuropsychiatric Aspects of HIV*. Geneva: WHO.

World Health Organization (1992) *The ICD-10 The International Classification of Diseases Classification of Mental and Behavioural Disorders* (10th revision) Geneva: WHO.

World Health Organization (1993) *The ICD-10 Classification of Mental and Behavioural Disorders: Diagnostic Criteria for Research*. Geneva: WHO.

Wright, N. and Lindesay, J. (1995) 'A survey of memory clinics in the British Isles.' *International Journal of Geriatric Psychiatry 1*, 10, 379–385.

Yale, R. (1995) *Developing Support Groups for Individuals with Early-Stage Alzheimer's Disease: Planning, Implementation and Evaluation*. Baltimore, MD: Health Professions Press.

Zoltan, B. (1996) *A Manual for the Treatment of Neuroimpaired Adults, 3rd Edition*. New York: Slack, Inc.

Zubaran, C., Fernando, J.G. and Rodnight, R. (1997) 'Wernicke-Korsakoff syndrome.' *Postgraduate Medical Journal 73*, 27–31.

Subject Index

Author Index